MEDICARE PART D PRESCRIPTION DRUG BENEFIT: A PRIMER

MEDICARE PART D PRESCRIPTION DRUG BENEFIT: A PRIMER

JENNIFER O'SULLIVAN

Novinka Books
New York

Copyright © 2008 by Nova Science Publishers, Inc.

All rights reserved. No part of this book may be reproduced, stored in a retrieval system or transmitted in any form or by any means: electronic, electrostatic, magnetic, tape, mechanical photocopying, recording or otherwise without the written permission of the Publisher.

For permission to use material from this book please contact us:
Telephone 631-231-7269; Fax 631-231-8175
Web Site: http://www.novapublishers.com

NOTICE TO THE READER

The Publisher has taken reasonable care in the preparation of this book, but makes no expressed or implied warranty of any kind and assumes no responsibility for any errors or omissions. No liability is assumed for incidental or consequential damages in connection with or arising out of information contained in this book. The Publisher shall not be liable for any special, consequential, or exemplary damages resulting, in whole or in part, from the readers' use of, or reliance upon, this material.

This publication is designed to provide accurate and authoritative information with regard to the subject matter covered herein. It is sold with the clear understanding that the Publisher is not engaged in rendering legal or any other professional services. If legal or any other expert assistance is required, the services of a competent person should be sought. FROM A DECLARATION OF PARTICIPANTS JOINTLY ADOPTED BY A COMMITTEE OF THE AMERICAN BAR ASSOCIATION AND A COMMITTEE OF PUBLISHERS.

LIBRARY OF CONGRESS CATALOGING-IN-PUBLICATION DATA
O'Sullivan, Jennifer.
Medicare Part D Prescription drug benefit : a primer / Jennifer O'Sullivan.
    p.;cm.
Includes bibliographical references and index.
ISBN 978-1-60456-622-2(softcover)
1.Insurance, Pharmaceutical services—Government policy—United States.2.Medicare. I.Title.[DNLM: 1. United States. Medicare Prescription Drug ,Improvement, and Modernization Act of 2003. 2.Medicare Part D—United States.3. Government Programs—United States. 4.insurance, Pharmaceutical services—United States. W 265 AA1 O85m 2008]
Ra412.3.O88   2008
36834'2600973—dc22   2008014850

Published by Nova Science Publishers, Inc. ✣ *New York.*

CONTENTS

Preface	vii
Overview	1
Enrollment in Part D	3
Part D Benefits	9
Special Provisions for Low-Income Populations	15
Part D Plans	25
Drug Payments	29
Plan Characteristics/ Beneficiary Protections	31
Payments to Plans	47
Beneficiary Premiums	53
Program Financing	55
Employer Subsidies	59
Issues	63
Key Part D Facts	67
References	77
Index	79

PREFACE[*]

The Medicare Prescription Drug, Improvement, and Modernization Act of 2003 (MMA, P.L.108-173) established a new voluntary prescription drug benefit under a new Medicare Part D, effective January 1, 2006. Prescription drug coverage is provided through private prescription drug plans (PDPs) or Medicare Advantage prescription drug (MA-PD) plans. Beneficiaries must enroll in one of these private plans in order to obtain their drug benefits. The program relies on these private plans to provide coverage and to bear some of the financial risk for drug costs; federal subsidies covering the bulk of the risk are provided to encourage participation.

At a minimum, plans offer "standard coverage" or alternative coverage with actuarially equivalent benefits. They may also offer enhanced benefits. All plans are required to meet certain minimum requirements, including those related to beneficiary protections. However, there are significant differences among plans in terms of benefit design, drugs included on plan formularies (i.e., list of covered drugs), cost-sharing applicable for particular drugs, and monthly premiums.

In general, beneficiaries can enroll in a plan, or change plan enrollment, when they first become eligible for Medicare or during the annual open enrollment period. The open enrollment period for 2008 is from November 15, 2007, to December 31, 2007. Plans can change from year to year. Beneficiary needs may also change. Therefore, beneficiaries should review their plan choice annually to make sure that their chosen plan continues to meet their needs.

A major focus of the drug benefit is the enhanced coverage provided to low-income individuals who enroll in Part D. Low-income enrollees,

---

[*] Excerpted from CRS report #RL34280, Updated December 7, 2007

including persons (known as "dual eligibles" — those persons enrolled in both Medicare and Medicaid) who previously received drug benefits under Medicaid, have their prescription drug costs paid under Part D. Persons with incomes below 150% of poverty have assistance with some portion of their premium and cost-sharing charges. Persons with the lowest incomes have the highest level of benefits. Dual-eligibles, as well as certain other low-income enrollees, are enrolled in plans with premiums at or below the low-income subsidy level for the region. They pay a zero premium for such plans (though they may select a plan with a higher premium and pay the difference). Some plans with premiums below the low-income subsidy level in 2007 will no longer qualify as zero premium plans in 2008. As a result, effective January 1, 2008, 1.6 million beneficiaries are being assigned to a new plan outside of their current organization, and an additional 965,000 are being assigned to a new plan with their current organization.

As of January 2007, approximately 23.9 million Medicare beneficiaries were enrolled in PDP and MA-PD plans. Of these, approximately 9.1 million were receiving low-income subsidy assistance. An additional 6.9 million beneficiaries had prescription drug coverage through a former employer that is receiving a federal subsidy for a portion of such coverage. Approximately 8.2 million beneficiaries had drug coverage through another source. An estimated 4.1 million or 10% of Medicare beneficiaries had no drug coverage.

OVERVIEW

The Medicare Prescription Drug, Improvement, and Modernization Act of 2003 (MMA, P.L.108-173) established a new voluntary prescription drug benefit under a new Medicare Part D. The new benefit was effective January 1, 2006. Prescription drug coverage is provided through private prescription drug plans (PDPs) or Medicare Advantage prescription drug (MA-PD) plans. At a minimum, these plans offer "standard coverage" or alternative coverage with actuarially equivalent benefits. Beneficiaries are required to enroll in one of these private plans in order to obtain their drug benefits. The program relies on these private plans to provide coverage and to bear some of the financial risk for drug costs; federal subsidies covering the bulk of the risk is provided to encourage participation.

Unlike other Medicare services, the benefits can only be obtained through private plans. Further, while all plans have to meet certain minimum requirements, there are significant differences among them in terms of benefit design, drugs included on plan formularies (i.e., list of covered drugs) and cost-sharing applicable for particular drugs.

A major focus of the drug benefit is the enhanced coverage provided to low-income individuals who enroll in Part D. Low-income enrollees, including persons (known as "dual eligibles" — those persons enrolled in both Medicare and Medicaid) who previously received drug benefits under Medicaid, have their prescription drug costs paid under Part D. Persons with incomes below 150% of poverty have assistance with some portion of their premium and cost-sharing charges. Persons with the lowest incomes have the highest level of benefits.

As of January 2007, approximately 23.9 million Medicare beneficiaries were enrolled in PDP and MA-PD plans. Of these, approximately 9.1 million were receiving low-income subsidy assistance. An additional 6.9 million beneficiaries had prescription drug coverage through a former employer that is receiving a federal subsidy for a portion of such coverage. Approximately 8.2 million beneficiaries had drug coverage through another source. An estimated 4.1 million or 10% of Medicare beneficiaries had no drug coverage.

ENROLLMENT IN PART D

All persons enrolled in Medicare Part A and/or Medicare Part B are eligible to enroll in a prescription drug plan under Part D. Beneficiaries enrolled in the "original Medicare" program obtain drug coverage through a PDP.

Beneficiaries enrolled in a managed care plan through a Medicare Advantage (MA) organization generally have to obtain drug coverage through their MA organization. If the MA enrollee wants to enroll in a PDP, he or she must drop their MA enrollment. There is one major exception to this rule. While most MA organizations are required to offer a MA-PD plan, private fee-for-service MA plans are not required to do so.[1] An individual enrolled in a plan not offering drug coverage may purchase coverage through a PDP.

PLAN INFORMATION

Different PDP and MA-PD plans are available in different parts of the country. Some organizations offer national plans. Information on plan availability and characteristics can be obtained from a number of sources. These include the Medicare toll-free information number (1-800-MEDICARE) and the website [http://www.medicare.gov]. Other organizations may also be able to provide assistance; these include State Health Insurance Assistance Programs (SHIPs) and other local organizations.

Beneficiaries must enroll with the organization offering their selected plan. They can enroll by mail, in person, or on the Web.

Beneficiaries (and persons assisting them) can look for a plan meeting their needs by going to the Medicare drug plan finder on [http://www.Medicare.gov]. An individual using the WEB tool should have a list of all the medications the beneficiary currently takes (together with dosage units). The plan finder will then show the beneficiary the five plans in the area with the lowest total annual cost for the package of drugs the individual takes. It is important to note that *a plan with the lowest premium and/or no deductible may not, in fact, be the lowest cost plan overall.* Further, the lowest cost plan for one member of a couple may not be the lowest cost plan for that person's spouse.

Beneficiaries should review their plan choice annually. Plans can make changes, effective January 1 each year. By October 31, of the previous year, plans are required to provide plan enrollees with a summary of the benefits for the following year and an outline of changes made from the current year. Plans can make a number of changes from one year to the next, including changing drugs included in the plan's formulary and/or changing the required cost-sharing charges for certain drugs. Therefore, enrollees should review materials provided by the plans to make sure that their chosen plans continue to meet their needs.

ENROLLMENT PERIODS

Initial Enrollment Period

In general, Medicare beneficiaries need to enroll in a plan during their initial enrollment period in order to avoid the delayed enrollment penalty. Persons on the Medicare rolls when the drug program began had until May 15, 2006 to enroll in a Part D plan for 2006.

Persons eligible for Medicare at a later date have an initial seven-month enrollment period beginning three months before the month of Medicare eligibility. This initial enrollment period is the same as that applicable for Medicare Part B. Coverage for these individuals begins on the first day of the first month following the month of enrollment, but no earlier than the first month they are entitled to Medicare.

Annual Open Enrollment Period

In general, an individual who does not enroll during their initial enrollment period is only able to enroll during the annual open enrollment period, which occurs from November 15-December 31 each year. Coverage begins the following January 1.

Creditable Coverage

Persons who fail to enroll during their initial enrollment period are subject to a penalty if they decide to enroll in Part D at a later date. However, they are not subject to the penalty if they have maintained "creditable" drug coverage through another public or private source. Creditable coverage is defined as drug benefits whose actuarial value equals or exceeds that of standard coverage. Sources of possible creditable coverage are retiree health coverage offered by a former employer or union and military coverage including TRICARE.

A beneficiary who has creditable coverage may wish to enroll in a Part D plan after the conclusion of their initial enrollment period. Care must be taken to assure that any noncoverage period between the two events does not exceed 63 days. Otherwise the beneficiary could be subject to a late enrollment penalty. For example, a retiree who is enrolled in a plan offered by his former employer decides in July 2008 that he wants to drop the employer coverage and enroll in Part D. The individual is not able to enroll in a Part D plan until the annual election period (November 15 to December 31). Coverage will not begin until the following January 1. He will probably want to keep his employer coverage through the end of 2008.

Special Enrollment Periods

In general, individuals can only enroll in Part D during their initial enrollment period or during the annual open enrollment period. However, there are a few limited occasions when an individual may have a special enrollment period including moving to a new geographic area, involuntary loss of creditable coverage; inadequate information provided on creditable coverage status, federal error, termination of a PDP contract, and plan failures. Special enrollment periods also apply for low-income enrollees deemed eligible for a subsidy outside of the initial or annual enrollment periods (See Low-Income discussion, below.)

Late Enrollment Penalty

The Part D delayed enrollment penalty provision is intended to prevent adverse selection. Adverse selection occurs when only those persons who think they need the benefit actually enroll in the program. When this happens, per capita costs are driven up, thereby causing more persons (presumably the healthier, and less costly ones) to drop out of the program. Over time, as more persons drop out, program costs become prohibitive. The intention of the penalty is to encourage all persons who do not have creditable coverage to enroll. Those who have creditable coverage are maintaining insurance protection and are not deferring coverage until they will actually need it.

The late enrollment penalty is assessed on persons who go for 63 days or longer after the close of their initial Part D enrollment period without creditable coverage and subsequently enroll in Part D. The penalty is based on the number of months the individual does not have creditable coverage. The premium that would otherwise apply is increased for each month without creditable coverage.

The late enrollment penalty is frequently described as being equal to at least 1% of the otherwise applicable premium for each uncovered month. The actual calculation is somewhat more complicated. The law specifies that the penalty is the greater of (1) the amount CMS determines is actuarially sound for each uncovered month or (2) 1% of the *base beneficiary premium* for each uncovered month. The "base beneficiary premium" is a national figure; it may therefore be different than the premium for the plan selected by the beneficiary. For uncovered months occurring during 2006 and 2007 the 1% calculation applies.

The penalty applies for as long as the individual is enrolled in Part D. The dollar amount of the each individual's penalty is expected to increase each year.

As noted above, individuals first eligible for Medicare on or before January 31, 2006, who failed to enroll by May 15, 2006, were not able to enroll until November 15, 2006, with coverage beginning January 1, 2007. If these individuals did not have creditable coverage during the period, they would have seven uncovered months. Their penalty would therefore be 7% of the base beneficiary premium — $1.91 (7% of the base monthly beneficiary premium of $27.35 for 2007). If these same persons waited an additional year, their penalty would be 19% of the base monthly beneficiary premium — $5.31 (19% of the base beneficiary premium of $27.93 for 2008).

Special rules apply for persons who qualify for the low-income subsidy outside of their initial enrollment period or the annual open enrollment period. These individuals can still enroll in a Part D plan throughout 2006, 2007, and 2008 and not be subject to the late enrollment penalty otherwise applicable to persons who miss the enrollment periods.

PART D BENEFITS

QUALIFIED COVERAGE

PDP sponsors and MA-PD plans are required to offer a minimum set of benefits, referred to as "qualified coverage." "Qualified coverage" is defined as either "standard prescription drug coverage" or "alternative prescription drug coverage" with at least actuarially equivalent benefits (i.e., having at least equivalent dollar value). In both cases, access must be provided to negotiated prices for drugs.

Defined Standard Coverage

Standard prescription drug coverage is defined as follows:

- *Deductible* paid by the beneficiary: $265 in 2007; $275 in 2008.
- 75% of costs paid by the program and 25% of costs paid by the beneficiary up to the *initial coverage limi*t: $2,400 in 2007 and $2,510 in 2008. (In 2007, this represents $798.75 in total out-of pocket costs paid by beneficiary and $2,400 in total spending; in 2008, this represents $833.75 in total out-of pocket costs paid by beneficiary and $2,510 in total spending.)
- 100% of costs paid by the beneficiary for drug spending falling in the *coverage gap up to the catastrophic threshold:* between $2,400.01 and $5,451.25 in 2007 and between $2510.01 and $5,726.25 in 2008 (In 2007, this represents $3850 in total out-of pocket costs paid by the beneficiary and $5,451.25 in total

spending; in 2008 this represents $4050 in total out-of pocket costs paid by the beneficiary and $5,726.25 in total spending).
- All costs paid by program over the "catastrophic" threshold or trigger ($5,451.25 in 2007, $5,726.25 in 2008) except for nominal beneficiary cost-sharing. Nominal cost-sharing is defined as the greater of (1) a copayment of $2.15 in 2007 ($2.25 in 2008) for generic drug or preferred multiple source drug and $5.35 in 2007 ($5.60 in 2008) for other drugs, or (2) 5% coinsurance.

Each year, the dollar amounts are increased by the annual percentage increase in average per capita aggregate expenditures for covered outpatient drugs for Medicare beneficiaries for the 12-month period ending in July of the previous year.

Table 1 shows the standard benefit as well as costs paid by low-income beneficiaries (discussed later in this report).

True Out-of-Pocket (TROOP) Costs

Beneficiaries must incur a certain level of out-of-pocket costs ($3,850 in 2007, $4,050 in 2008) before catastrophic protection begins. Costs are only considered incurred if they are incurred for the deductible, cost-sharing, or benefits not paid because they fall in the coverage gap (sometimes referred to as the *doughnut hole*). Incurred costs do not include amounts for which no benefits are provided because a drug is excluded under a particular plan's formulary. Costs are treated as incurred, and thus treated as true out-of-pocket (*TROOP*) costs only if they are paid by the individual (or by another family member on behalf of the individual), paid on behalf of a low-income individual under the subsidy provisions, or under a state pharmaceutical assistance program. Any costs for which the individual is reimbursed by insurance or otherwise do not count toward the TROOP amount.

Table 1. Part D Standard Benefits, 2007 and 2008
(by per capita drug spending category)

			Subsidy Eligible Individuals[a]			
	All beneficiaries		Full Subsidy Eligible		Other Subsidy Eligible	
Total drug spending (dollar ranges)	Paid by Part D	Paid by enrollee	Paid by Part D	Paid by enrollee	Paid by Part D	Paid by enrollee
$0 up to Deductible ($265 in 2007 $275 in 2008)	0%	$265 in 2007 $275 in 2008	$265 in 2007 $275 in 2008	0	$212 in 2007 $219 in 2008	$53 in 2007 $56 in 2008
Between Deductible and **Initial Coverage Limit** $265.01-$2,400 in 2007 $275.01-$2,510 in 2008	75%	25%	100% less enrollee cost-sharing	Institutionalized duals: $0 Duals under 100% of poverty: $1/$3.10 in 2007[c] $1.05/$3.10 in 2008[c] Others: $2.15/$5.35 in 2007[d] $2.25/5.60 in 2008[d]	85%	15%
Between Initial Coverage Limit and **Catastrophic Trigger** ($2,400.01-$5,451.25 in 2007 $2,510.01-$5,726.25 in 2008)	0%	100%	100% less enrollee cost-sharing	Institutionalized duals: $0 Duals under 100% of poverty: $1/$3.10[c] $1.05/$3.10 in 2008[c] Others: $2.15/$5.35 in 2007[d] $2.25/$5.60 in 2008[d]	85%	15%
Over catastrophic trigger ($5,451.26 and over in 2007 $5,726.26 and over in 2008)	95%[b]	5%[e]	100%	0	100% less enrollee cost-sharing	$2.15/$5.35 in 2007d $2.25/$5.60 in 2008d

Source: CMS, Notification of Changes in Medicare Part D Payment for Calendar Year 2008 (Part D Payment Notification), Memo to PDP Sponsors, MA organizations and other Interested parties, April 2, 2007.

a. Subsidy eligible persons are low-income individuals entitled to assistance with Part D premiums and cost-sharing. Full-subsidy eligible individuals can enroll in plans for which they pay no premiums; other subsidy eligible individuals can enroll in plans for which a portion of their premiums are subsidized. Both groups have assistance with otherwise applicable cost-sharing charges.
b. Assumes enrollee has met true out-of-pocket (TROOP) threshold of $3,850 in 2007, $4,050 in 2008.
c. $1 in 2007 ($1.05 in 2008) per prescription for generic or preferred drugs that are multiple source drugs; $3.10 per prescription for other drugs.
d. $2.15 in 2007 ($2.25 in 2008) per prescription for generic or preferred drugs that are multiple source drugs; $5.35 ($5.60) per prescription for other drugs.
e. Copayment amounts apply if larger.

Actuarially Equivalent Plans

Plans may offer actuarially equivalent coverage, providing they meet certain requirements. These plans have the same actuarial value as the standard benefit, but a different benefit structure. For example, they may eliminate the deductible, but have cost-sharing requirements higher than the 25% amount under basic standard coverage. They may also used tiered cost-sharing under which generics have the lowest cost-sharing, preferred brands have the next level of cost sharing and nonpreferred brand have higher cost sharing requirements. Some plans may have a specialty tier for very high cost drugs.

CMS recognizes two types of actuarially equivalent plans. Plans labeled "actuarially equivalent standard" offer a different cost-sharing structure. Plans labeled "basic alternative standard" may reduce the deductible, change cost-sharing, and/or change the initial coverage limit. In 2007, 51% of enrollees are in plans offering actuarially equivalent benefits.

Enhanced Coverage

Plans may offer enhanced coverage which exceeds the value of defined standard coverage. This coverage includes both basic coverage and supplemental benefits. Supplemental benefits may include some coverage in the coverage gap (for example coverage of generic drugs) and/or reductions in cost-sharing that increase the actuarial value of the package. In 2007, 35% of enrollees were in plans offering enhanced coverage.

A PDP-sponsor cannot offer an enhanced plan unless it also offers a basic plan in the service area. As noted above, MA organizations offering MA coordinated care plans are required to offer at least one plan in the service area with drug coverage. The drug coverage can be either basic coverage or enhanced coverage with no premium for the supplemental benefits.[2]

Access to Negotiated Prices

All plans are required to provide beneficiaries with access to negotiated prices for covered Part D drugs. This access must be provided even when no Part D benefits are payable because the beneficiary has not met the deductible or the beneficiary is in the coverage gap. Negotiated prices are to take into account negotiated price concessions for covered drugs that are passed through to enrollees at the point of sale. Such price concessions include discounts, direct or indirect subsidies, rebates, and other direct or indirect remunerations.

SPECIAL PROVISIONS FOR LOW-INCOME POPULATIONS

A major focus of Part D is the enhanced coverage provided to low-income individuals. Persons with incomes below 150% of poverty (and assets below specified levels) have assistance with some portion of Part D premium and cost-sharing charges. Persons with the lowest incomes have the highest level of assistance.

ELIGIBILITY FOR LOW-INCOME SUBSIDY (LIS) ASSISTANCE

Definition of Eligible Groups

Special premium and cost-sharing subsidies are available for low-income persons. This population is divided into two main groups with the first group divided into subgroups for purposes of determining cost-sharing requirements. The two main groups are defined as follows:

"Full Subsidy Eligible Individuals"

This group includes all persons who (1) are enrolled in a PDP plan or MA-PD plan; (2) have incomes below 135% of the federal poverty level ($13,783 for an individual and $18,481 for a couple in 2007); and (3) have resources in 2007 below $6,120 for an individual and $9,190 for a couple (increased each year by the percentage increase in the consumer price index, or CPI). The 2007 resource limits are generally publicized as $7,620 and $12,190 because $1,500 per person is excluded for burial expenses.

The following groups of persons are also defined as full subsidy eligible individuals:

- *Dual Eligibles.* These are persons entitled to the full range of benefits under their state's Medicaid program. Prior to January 1, 2006, these persons received their drug benefits under Medicaid. Effective January 1, 2006, their drug benefits are provided through Part D. All full benefit dual eligible individuals are deemed to be in the full subsidy eligible group, regardless of whether they meet the other eligibility requirements.
- Recipients of Supplemental Security Income (SSI) benefits; or
- *Enrollees in a Medicare Savings Program (MSP).* MMA permitted the Secretary to extend full subsidy eligible coverage to enrollees in MSP. (Implementing regulations extended coverage to this group). There are three Medicare Savings programs that provide Medicaid assistance for Medicare premiums and cost-sharing charges. The three groups are (1) qualified Medicare beneficiaries (QMBs),[3] (2) specified low-income Medicare beneficiaries (SLMBs),[4] and (3) qualifying individuals (QI-1s).[5]

"Other Subsidy Eligible Individuals"

This group includes all other persons who (1) are enrolled in a PDP plan or MA-PD plan, (2) have incomes below 150% of poverty ($15,315 for an individual and $20,535 for a couple in 2007), and (3) have resources in 2007 below $10,210 for an individual and $20,410 for a couple (increased in future years by the percentage increase in the CPI). The publicized resource limits of $11,710 and $23,410 include a $1,500 per person burial allowance.

Definition of Income and Assets

The definitions of income and assets generally follows that used for determining eligibility under the QMB, SLMB, and QI-1 programs (which in turn link back to the definitions used for purposes of the SSI program). There are, however, a few items that should be noted:

Special Provisions for Low-Income Populations

- *Family Size.* Currently, the federal poverty level (FPL) used for income determinations is that applicable for an individual or for a couple. MMA specified that the FPL is to be that for the family of the size involved. Therefore, the regulations define the family size to include, in addition to the applicant and spouse, additional persons related to the applicant who live in the same residence and depend on the applicant or spouse for at least one-half of their financial support. The income of these additional persons would not, however, be used in the determination of eligibility.
- *Resources.* MMA provides for the development of a simplified application in which applicants attest to their level of resources and submit minimal documentation. Only liquid resources (or those that could be converted to cash within 20 days) and real estate that is not the applicant's primary residence are considered. Liquid resources include such things as checking and savings accounts, stocks, and bonds. Vehicles are excluded because they are not considered liquid assets.
- *More Generous State Standards.* The law (Section 1902(r)(2) of the Social Security Act) allows states to use more generous income and assets rules for determining eligibility for the QMB, SLMB, and QI-1 programs. A few states have elected this option. As noted above, MMA permitted the Secretary to include all persons meeting

QMB, SLMB, and QI-1 criteria in the full subsidy eligible group; the Secretary elected to do so. However, only persons on QMB, SLMB, or QI-1 rolls are actually included. States are not permitted to use the less restrictive methodologies for other subsidy eligibility determinations; the standards will be the same nationwide for these persons.

LIS BENEFITS

Subsidies are provided for both premiums and cost-sharing charges.

Premium Subsidies

Premium subsidies are available for both full subsidy eligible and other subsidy eligible persons. However, the amount of assistance is less for the second group.

Full Subsidy Eligible Individuals

All full subsidy-eligible individuals receive a premium subsidy equal to 100% of the low-income benchmark premium amount (see following discussion), but in no case higher than the actual premium amount for basic coverage under the plan selected by the enrollee.

In addition, the premium subsidy amount can not be less than the premium for the lowest-cost PDP plan in the region. Thus, all full subsidy eligible individuals are entitled to a full premium subsidy for at least one plan in their region. However, if a beneficiary selects a plan with a premium higher than the benchmark, the beneficiary is liable for the additional costs.

Full subsidy eligible individuals, but not other subsidy eligible individuals, also have a premium subsidy for any Part D late enrollment penalty equal to 80% for the first 60 months of delayed enrollment and 100% thereafter.

Other Subsidy Eligible Individuals

All other subsidy eligible individuals have a sliding scale premium subsidy ranging from 100% of the premium subsidy amount at 135% of poverty to 0% of such value at 150% of poverty. Specifically, the subsidy is 75% for persons with incomes above 135% but at or below 140% of poverty, 50% for persons with incomes above 140% but at or below 145% of poverty; and 25% for persons with incomes above 145% but below 150% of poverty.

Calculation of Low-Income Benchmark Premium

The low-income benchmark premium for a region is the weighted average of the monthly beneficiary premiums for basic prescription drug coverage. The low-income benchmark is defined as the weighted average premium, with the weight based on plan enrollment. For 2006, the program's first year, all PDPs were assigned an equal weight. (MAs were enrollment weighted if they had 2005 enrollment.)

Beginning in 2007, the bid amounts were to be weighted by plan enrollment in the previous year. However, since many beneficiaries selected low-cost plans in 2006, using a weighted average would have the effect of reducing the regional low-income benchmark premium amounts. Instead, CMS decided to transition to the weighting methodology using the Secretary's demonstration authority ("Medicare Demonstration to Transition Enrollment of Low-Income Subsidy Beneficiaries").

For 2007, it used the same methodology used for 2006. Beginning for 2008, it is implementing a transition from the 2006 methodology and the weighted average method based on actual plan enrollments. In 2008, 50% of the regional benchmark is based on the 2006 averaging methodology and 50% on the enrollment-weighted average. For determining the enrollment-weighted average, Part D enrollees in PDPs and MA-PDs in June 2007 are used. **Table 2** shows the applicable 2008 amount by PDP region.

Table 2. Low-Income Benchmark, by Region, 2008

Region	State(s)	Monthly Subsidy	Region	State(s)	Monthly Subsidy
1	NH, ME	$30.64	18	MO	$26.71
2	CT, MA, RI, VT	29.17	19	AR	27.69
3	NY	24.18	20	MS	31.35
4	NJ	31.23	21	LA	24.62
5	DE, DC, MD	30.78	22	TX	25.01
6	PA, WV	26.59	23	OK	28.04
7	VA	31.03	24	KS	30.62
8	NC	33.43	25	IA, MN, MT, ND, NE, SD, WY	30.61
9	SC	31.12	26	NM	19.28
10	GA	30.04	27	CO	24.59
11	FL	19.16	28	AZ	15.92
12	AL, TN	28.29	29	NV	16.64
13	MI	30.49	30	OR, WA	30.19
14	OH	26.82	31	ID, UT	33.53
15	IN, KY	33.50	32	CA	19.80
16	WI	31.03	33	HI	24.32
17	IL	30.26	34	AK	36.42

Source: CMS, at [http://www.cms.hhs.gov/MedicareAdvtgSpecRateStats/RSD/list.asp#TopOfPage].

Cost-Sharing Subsidies

Cost-sharing subsides are linked to "standard prescription drug coverage." Full subsidy eligibles have no deductible, no coverage gap (i.e., no "doughnut hole"), and no cost-sharing over the catastrophic threshold. Full benefit dual eligibles who are residents of a medical institution or nursing facility have no cost-sharing. Other full benefit dual eligible individuals with incomes up to 100% of poverty have cost-sharing, for all costs up to the out-of-pocket threshold, of $1 in 2007 ($1.05 in 2008) for a generic drug prescription or preferred multiple source drug prescription and $3.10 (in both 2007 and 2008) for any other drug prescription. All other full subsidy eligible individuals have cost-sharing, for all costs up to the out-of-pocket threshold, of $2.15 in 2007 ($2.25 in 2008) for a generic drug or preferred multiple source drug and $5.35 in 2007 ($5.60 in 2008) for any other drug. (See **Table 1**.)

Other subsidy eligible individuals have a $53 deductible in 2007 ($56 in 2008), 15% coinsurance for all costs up to the catastrophic trigger level, and cost-sharing for costs above this level of $2.15 in 2007 ($2.25 in 2008) for a generic drug prescription or preferred multiple source drug prescription and $5.35 in 2007 ($5.60 in 2008) for any other drug prescription. (See **Table 1**.)

Each year, the cost-sharing amounts for full benefit dual eligibles below 100% of poverty are increased by the increase in the CPI. The cost-sharing amounts for all other persons, and the deductible amount for other subsidy eligible individuals, are increased by the annual percentage increase in per capita beneficiary expenditures for Part D covered drugs.

ENROLLMENT

Generally there is a two-step process for low-income persons to gain Part D coverage. First, a determination must be made that they qualify for the assistance; and, second, they must enroll, or be enrolled, in a specific Part D plan. Special procedures were established to make the process easier. The procedures are different for different categories of low-income enrollees.

Dual Eligibles

There were more than 6 million dual eligibles who needed to be enrolled in a Part D plan, effective January 1, 2006. CMS established an auto-enrollment process which was intended to assure there was no gap in coverage, though the program did encounter some problems in the early stages.

The auto-enrollment process was random among plans with premiums at or below the low-income benchmark premium. Persons becoming dually eligible after January 2006 are also auto-enrolled into a Part D plan.

There are a number of differences among available plans. Key differences are drugs included in plan formularies and pharmacies participating in the plan as network pharmacies. Some dual eligibles may find that they are auto-enrolled in a plan which may not best meet their needs. For this reason, they are able to change enrollment at any time with the new coverage effective the following month. It should be noted that if an enrollee selects a plan with a premium above the low-income benchmark, he or she is required to pay the difference.

Enrollees in Medicare Savings Program

CMS established a process, labeled "facilitated enrollment" for enrollees in Medicare Savings programs (MSPs), SSI enrollees, and persons who applied for and were approved for low-income subsidy assistance. The basic features applicable to auto-enrollment for dual eligibles (i.e., random assignment to plans with premiums below the low-income benchmark and assignment of MA enrollees to the lowest-cost MA-PD plan offered by the MA organization) were extended to facilitate enrollment.

Beneficiaries eligible for facilitated enrollment in 2006 were sent notices informing them of the plans they would be enrolled in if they took no action. If the beneficiary failed to select another plan (and did not decline Part D enrollment), he or she was considered to have enrolled in the assigned plan, effective May 1, 2006. Facilitated enrollment also applies for persons becoming eligible for MSP after that date. As is the case for a dual eligible, an MSP enrollee can change plan enrollment throughout the year.

Other Low-Income Persons

MMA extended low-income subsidies to all persons with incomes below 150% of poverty and assets below specified levels. Persons not identified as dual eligibles, MSP enrollees, or SSI recipients may qualify, but they need to submit an application. The Social Security Administration (SSA) generally makes eligibility determinations for those who fill out the applications, though an individual may request the state Medicaid agency to make the determination.

CMS facilitates enrollment in Part D plans for persons identified as qualifying for extra help. However, unless they are dual eligibles or MSP enrollees, they are only able to switch plans once during the year, with the new coverage effective the following month.

2008 Enrollment

There are several circumstances under which a low-income subsidy-eligible person will experience a change from 2007 to 2008. These include cases in which an individual (1) is enrolled in a plan whose 2008 premium will no longer fall below the low-income benchmark premium, (2) is enrolled in a plan that terminates its participation in Part D, (3) loses automatic eligibility for the low-income subsidy in 2008, or (4) falls into a different subsidy category.

Individuals Enrolled in Plans that no Longer Have Premiums Below the Benchmark or in Plans that Terminate

CMS has established a process for reassigning these beneficiaries to a different Part D plan. Beneficiaries to be reassigned must meet all of the following criteria:

- They were deemed eligible for a subsidy in 2007 because they were dual eligibles, participants in MSP, SSI recipients, or because they applied and were found eligible for the full subsidy.
- They will continue to be eligible for a subsidy in 2008.
- They were originally auto-enrolled or had their enrollment facilitated into a PDP.
- They did not elect to enroll in a different plan.
- Their current plan has a 2008 premium that is above the "de minimus amount" (which is the benchmark plus $1) or is terminating at the end of 2007.

Beneficiaries meeting all of these criteria will be reassigned to a different PDP in the region as follows. The beneficiaries will be assigned to another plan in the same region offered by the same PDP sponsor, if the sponsor has a plan with a premium at or below the benchmark (or, if there is none available, a plan below the de minimus amount). If no such plan exists, CMS will randomly assign beneficiaries among PDP sponsors with at least one plan with a premium at or below the benchmark. CMS will notify beneficiaries in early November 2007 of their plan assignment; they will be reassigned to a new plan effective January 1, 2008. However, beneficiaries may voluntarily elect to stay in their current plan (if it is still offered) or select a different plan from the one assigned by CMS. If they wish to select a new plan, they should do so by December 7, 2007, so that their assignment to the new plan can be processed on a timely basis.

Beneficiaries who changed plans after they were either auto-assigned to a plan or had their enrollment facilitated into a plan will not have their selection changed by CMS. However, they will be informed that their plan's premium is rising above the regional low-income subsidy amount by more than the de minimus $1 in 2008 and will therefore be liable for any excess if they stay with their current plan. The beneficiary is free to change his or her selection.

On October 29, 2007, CMS announced that it was sending reassignment notices to 1.6 million persons who would be reassigned to a new plan outside of their current organization and an additional 965,000 persons who were to be reassigned to a new plan within their current organization. It also announced that it was sending "chooser notices" to the 442,000 persons who qualified for a full premium subsidy but the 2007 plan they had selected would have a premium in 2008 above the de minimus amount.

Individuals Losing Automatic Eligibility for Low-Income Subsidy.

Persons automatically qualifying for a low-income subsidy are dual eligibles, persons enrolled in MSP, and SSI recipients. In September 2007, CMS sent letters to those beneficiaries losing their automatic eligibility for a low-income subsidy in 2008 because they no longer fall into one of these categories. At the same time, these beneficiaries were told they still might qualify for assistance and were encouraged to file a low-income subsidy application with SSA. The application and a postage-paid envelope were enclosed with each notice.

Individuals Falling into a Different Subsidy Category

Beneficiaries who will experience a change in their low-income subsidy level in 2008 received a notice in October 2007 informing them of the change. These beneficiaries will be subject to different cost-sharing requirements.

INTERACTION WITH STATE PHARMACY ASSISTANCE PROGRAMS

A number of states have had state pharmaceutical assistance programs (SPAPs) in place for a number of years. These programs were set up to offer prescription drug benefits to low-income individuals who did not have Medicaid drug coverage. Many, but not all, persons enrolled in SPAPs are eligible for low-income subsidies under Part D. SPAP payments made on their behalf to cover Part D cost-sharing charges count toward the individual's true out-of-pocket (TROOP) costs trigger.

MMA defines an SPAP as one that provides assistance to persons in all Part D plans and does not discriminate based on the Part D plan in which the individual is enrolled. CMS interpreted the Part D language to mean that if an SPAP offers Part D premium assistance or supplemental Part D cost-sharing assistance, it must offer equal assistance for all PDP and MA-PD plans available in the region, and may not steer beneficiaries to one plan or another through benefit design or otherwise. Violation of this nondiscrimination rule would violate the SPAP's status with respect to counting TROOP. The inability to steer beneficiaries to a selected plan or plans effectively meant that an SPAP could not auto-enroll its participants in preferred Part D plans. This proved to be a concern for some states who argued they should be able to enroll their beneficiaries in preferred plans if they gave individuals the option to switch to other plans if they wanted to.

CMS established policies intended to balance the need to adhere to the nondiscrimination requirement with state concerns. It generally required SPAPs to provide wrap-around benefits (namely fill in the gaps) for their Part D beneficiaries regardless of the plan the beneficiary chose to enroll in and permitted SPAPS (when acting as authorized representatives) to enroll their beneficiaries in Part D plans using only beneficiary-specific criteria to limit the selection of part D plans. In its 2008 call letter to plans, CMS refined the policy to explicitly permit states to adopt reasonable coordinating criteria. SPAPs with authorized representative status are allowed to facilitate enrollment of their beneficiaries into plans that agree to the state-specific coordination criteria (such as offering similar formularies and pharmacy network structures). Such criteria must be of the kind that any Part D plan could meet if it chose. SPAPs must continue to permit beneficiaries who wish to enroll in a plan not meeting the coordinating criteria to do so; they must provide the same wrap-around benefits or assistance.

PART D PLANS

PDP REGIONS

MMA required the Secretary to designate PDP regions. The service area for a PDP plan must include the entire PDP region. A plan can be offered in more than one PDP region, including all PDP regions.

The Secretary designated 34 PDP regions. No region is smaller than a state. Twenty-five states are individual regions. Twelve states are part of two state regions. There is one region with two states and the District of Columbia, one region with four states, and one region with seven states. (See **Table 2** for states in each region.)

APPROVAL OF PDP PLANS

Each year, CMS issues a call letter to contractors planning to offer PDP and/or MA plans in the coming year. The 2008 call letter issued in April 2007, combined contracting guidance for both programs. Potential PDP and MA sponsors are required to submit bids by the first Monday in June of the previous year. Each potential PDP sponsor is required to submit a bid and supplemental information for each Part D plan it intends to offer. The following information is to be included with the bid: (1) the coverage to be provided; (2) actuarial value of qualified prescription drug coverage in the region for a beneficiary with a national average risk profile; (3) information on the bid including the basis for the actuarial value, the portion of the bid attributable to basic coverage and, if applicable, the portion attributable to enhanced coverage, and assumptions regarding the reinsurance subsidy (see discussion on financing, below); and (4) service area.

CMS reviews the information to conduct negotiations regarding the terms and conditions of the proposed bid and benefit plan. Private fee-for-service plans under Medicare Part C are exempt from the negotiation requirements.

MMA specified that the negotiating authority is similar to the authority the Director of the Office of Personnel Management has with respect to Federal Employees Health Benefits (FEHB) plans. However, the law specifically states that the Secretary may not interfere with the negotiations between drug manufacturers and pharmacies and PDP sponsors. Further, the Secretary may not require a particular formulary or institute a price structure for the reimbursement of covered Part D drugs. This is known as the "non-interference provision."

CMS can only approve a plan if certain requirements are met. The plan must comply with Part D requirements, including those relating to beneficiary protections. CMS must determine that the plan and the sponsor meet requirements relating to actuarial determinations. Further, the Secretary may not find that the design of the plan and its benefits (including any formulary and tiered formulary structure) are likely to discourage enrollment by certain beneficiaries.

For both 2007 and 2008, CMS negotiated with plan sponsors to ensure that each bid submitted represented a meaningful variation based on plan characteristics that would provide beneficiaries with substantially different options. CMS has stated that it would not expect that more than two bids from a sponsoring organization would provide meaningful variation unless one of the bids is an enhanced alternative plan with coverage in the gap.

CONTRACTS

The law and regulations establish requirements for PDP plan sponsors. In general, a PDP sponsor must be licensed under state law as a risk bearing entity eligible to offer health insurance or health benefits coverage in each state in which it is offering a drug plan. (Alternatively, it could meet solvency standards established by CMS for entities not licensed by the state.) The entity must assume its financial risk on a prospective basis for covered benefits; it may obtain insurance (i.e., reinsure) or make other arrangements for the costs of coverage.

PDP sponsors enter into contracts with CMS. The contract may cover more than one Part D plan. Under terms of the contract, the sponsor agrees to comply with Part D requirements and have satisfactory administrative and management arrangements.

CMS cannot enter a contract with an organization unless it meets minimum enrollment requirements of 5,000 individuals (or 1,500 individuals if the organization primarily serves individuals residing outside of urbanized areas). CMS may waive the minimum enrollment requirement during the first contract year for a sponsor in a region.

Each contract is for a period of 12 months. An entity is determined qualified to renew its contract annually only if CMS informs the entity that it is qualified to renew the contract and the plan sponsor has not provided CMS of a notice of its intent not to renew. However, renewal of a contract is contingent on reaching agreement on the bid. If the sponsor and CMS cannot reach agreement, no renewal takes place.

PLAN MONITORING

CMS monitors plan operations with particular emphasis on the following five performance measures: telephone customer service wait times; frequency and types of complaints; timeliness and resolution of appeals; completeness of enrollment information available to pharmacists; and the percent of drug pricing changes available on the drug plan finder on the WEB and the percent of drugs on the finder with price increases.

DRUG PAYMENTS

Part D plan sponsors (or the pharmaceutical benefit managers (PBMs) they have contracted with) negotiate prices with drug manufacturers, wholesalers and pharmacies. The negotiated price (i.e., the price that is available to the beneficiary) is net of some or all of rebates, discounts and other price concessions. The plan's negotiated price may reflect the same prices that a health plan or PBM would get for its commercially insured members or it may be different.

Part D plans are expected to negotiate on behalf of enrollees for price discounts. These discounts may be passed on to beneficiaries and the program in many ways including lower copayment and coinsurance, lower prices (compared with retail prices), and lower premiums. A portion of the manufacturers price concessions may be retained by the plan.

Plan sponsors negotiate with pharmacies in order to include a sufficient number and geographic distribution of pharmacies in their networks. The plan reimburses the pharmacy for the cost of the drug, plus a dispensing fee. Pharmacies set their own rates for dispensing drugs but may give the plan a discount on their usual rate.

A plan's negotiated prices may be found on the www.medicare.gov website. Beneficiaries can also compare negotiated prices for different plans in their area. By law, the net prices charged to Part D plans are not made public. The amount of price concessions is reported to CMS.

The 2007 Medicare trustees report estimated that plans achieved an average savings of 21% from retail discounts and utilization management in 2006. This savings level was estimated to increase to 22% in 2007 where it was expected to remain through 2016. It further reported that the average rebate was estimated by plans to be 5.2% in 2006 and 4.6% in 2007; it was expected to remain at about 4%-5% through 2015. The report noted that these figures were averages; generics typically do not carry rebates, while brand name drugs may carry rebates as high as 20-30%. As noted above, some but not necessarily all, of these savings may be passed on to beneficiaires.

PLAN CHARACTERISTICS/ BENEFICIARY PROTECTIONS

The law and regulations establish requirements that plans must meet.

MARKETING/BENEFICIARY COMMUNICATIONS

Plan sponsors are required to assure timely and accurate information in their marketing materials. Such materials must be approved by CMS. In its 2008 call letter to plans, CMS emphasized that organizations are responsible for the actions of sales agents/brokers whether they are employed or contracted. It stated that organizations must assure that these individuals are properly trained in both Medicare and the details of the products being offered. Plan sponsors must provide strong oversight of marketing activities.

Employees of an organization or independent agents or brokers acting on behalf of the organization may not solicit Medicare beneficiaries door-to-door. They must first ask permission before providing assistance in a beneficiary's home, prior to conducting any sales representations or accepting an enrollment form in person.

Plan sponsors are required to provide enrollees with an evidence of coverage (EOC) document upon enrollment and annually thereafter. The EOC gives the details about how the plan works, covered benefits and related cost-sharing responsibilities. Plans are also required to provide current enrollees with an annual notice of change (ANOC) document, showing changes for the forthcoming year, prior to the annual open enrollment period. The ANOC does not provide a list of drugs added or deleted from the formulary or drugs whose tier has changed. It does however note if such changes have been made.

For the 2008 plan year, plan sponsors were encouraged to use a combined model ANOC/EOC document to be forwarded to beneficiaries by October 31, 2007; in addition they were required to mail information on plan formularies. Alternatively, plans could use a separate ANOC and statement of benefits, with the EOC to follow by January 31, 2008.

In its draft 2008 call letter, CMS had considered allowing plan comparisons of MA and PDPs in a specific service area. However, CMS stated that based on negative response to the proposal, it was persuaded that it was not practical or meaningful to develop a comparison that was not beneficiary specific.

As noted earlier, beneficiaries can obtain targeted information about plans by using the Medicare prescription drug plan finder tool on the www.medicare.gov website. Information for 2008, was posted October 11, 2007.

COVERED DRUGS

In order for a drug to be paid under Part D, it must be a drug that can be included under Part D. Further, it must be included in the formulary of the individual's Part D plan.

Covered Drugs

The law defines covered Part D drugs as (1) outpatient prescription drugs approved by the Food and Drug Administration (FDA), and used for a medically accepted indication; (2) biological products which may only be dispensed upon a prescription and which are licensed under the Public Health Service (PHS) Act and produced at a licensed establishment; (3) insulin (including medical supplies associated with the injection of insulin); and (4) vaccines licensed under the PHS Act. Also included are drugs treated as being included in a plan's formulary as a result of a coverage determination or appeal.

Excluded Drugs

The law specifically excludes drugs which may be excluded from coverage under Medicaid, except for drugs used for smoking cessation. This exclusion applies to (1) benzodiazepines; (2) barbiturates; (3) drugs used for anorexia, weight loss, or weight gain; (4) fertility drugs; (5) drugs used for cosmetic purposes or hair growth; (6) drugs for symptomatic relief for coughs and colds; (7) prescription vitamins and minerals; and (8) covered drugs when the manufacturer requires, as a condition of sale, that associated tests be purchased exclusively from the manufacturer. In addition, drugs which are used for the treatment of sexual or erectile dysfunction are excluded, unless they are used to treat another condition for which the drug has been approved by the FDA (off label uses for these drugs are not covered).

It should be noted that a Part D sponsor may elect to include one or more of these drugs in an enhanced Part D plan. However, no federal subsidy is available for the associated costs.

Part B Versus Part D

Part D will not pay for drugs which are covered under Part B (even if the individual is not actually enrolled in Part B). Some drugs and vaccines can potentially be covered under both Part B or Part D. In this case a determination must be made as to whether or not the drug can be covered under Part B in the particular case. Part B covered drugs include drugs which are not usually self-administered and provided incident to a physicians's professional services; immunosuppressive drugs for persons who have had a Medicare-covered transplant; erythropoietin for persons with end stage renal disease; oral anti-cancer drugs; drugs requiring administration via a nebulizer or infusion pump in the home; and certain vaccines (influenza, pneumococcal, and hepatitis B for intermediate or high risk persons).

Vaccine Administration

Beginning in 2008, Part D plans (not Part B) are required to cover the costs for the administration of Part D covered vaccines.

Physicians will need to bill the patients for these services; the patient will then need to bill the Part D plan.

FORMULARIES

Part D formularies are required to meet a number of specific requirements.

Pharmacy and Therapeutic (P&T) Committee

A P&T committee must develop and review the formulary. A majority of the members must be practicing physicians, practicing pharmacists or both. Further, they must come from clinical specialties that adequately represent the needs of beneficiaries.

The committee, when developing and reviewing the formulary, is to base clinical decisions on the strength of scientific evidence and standards of practice. It should also take into account whether including a particular drug in the formulary (or in a particular tier in the formulary) has therapeutic value in terms of safety and efficacy.

Minimum Requirements

The formulary must include drug categories and classes that cover all disease states. MMA required CMS to request the United States Pharmacopeia (USP) to develop a list of categories and classes which may be used by plans and to periodically revise such classification as appropriate. Part D plans that use a classification system that is consistent with the USP classification system are deemed to satisfy a safe harbor and will be approved by CMS. CMS will review systems of plans proposing to adopt an alternative classification to determine if it is similar to the USP or other commonly used system.

A plan's formulary must include at least two drugs in each category or class (unless only one drug is available in the category or class, or two drugs are available but one drug is clinically superior). The two drug requirement must be met through the provision of two chemically distinct drugs. Plans cannot meet the requirement by including only two dosage forms or strengths of the same drug or a brand name and its generic equivalent. However, CMS does expect plans to include multiple strengths and dosage forms where available.

Six Classes of Clinical Concern

Part D plans are required to cover all, or substantially all of the drugs in the following six drug categories: immunosuppressant, antidepressant, antipsychotic, anticonvulsant, antiretroviral, and antineoplastic. CMS instituted this policy to mitigate the risks and complications associated with an interruption of therapy for vulnerable populations. For 2008, the requirement applies to drugs available on April 16, 2007. New drugs or newly approved drugs within these six classes that come into the market at a later date will be subject to expedited P&T committee review.

Plan sponsors cannot implement prior authorization or step therapy requirements that are intended to steer beneficiaries to preferred alternatives within these classes for beneficiaries currently taking a drug. For beneficiaries beginning treatment in these categories, such management techniques may be used for categories other than HIV/AIDS drugs.

CMS Review

CMS reviews and approves drug lists that are consistent with best practice formularies currently in widespread use. It reviews formularies for at least one drug in each of the USP Formulary Key Drug Types. It reviews tier placement to provide assurance that the formulary does not substantially discourage enrollment of certain beneficiaries. It analyzes formularies to determine whether appropriate access is afforded to drugs or drug classes addressed in widely accepted treatment guidelines which are indicative of general best practice. It also analyzes the availability and tier position of the most commonly prescribed drug classes for the general Medicare population and the dually eligible population. CMS also looks to existing best practices to check plans' use of utilization management tools such as prior authorization, quantity limits and step therapy (where a lower cost drug is first tried before a higher cost drug may be used).

For the 2008 contract year, CMS stated that it was expanding its review of drugs commonly used by the dual eligible population to 200 and incorporating the top 100 drugs used in the Medicare drug discount card program (the temporary program for the low-income persons in place in 2004-2005). It was also expanding the number of treatment guidelines to ensure best practice drugs are included in the formulary. Finally, it would use the presence of USP Formulary Key Drug Types as an outlier test to ensure these drugs are strongly represented on all Part D formularies.

Specialty Tier

A Part D plan is allowed to exempt a formulary tier in which it places very high cost and unique items from tiered cost-sharing exceptions. In order to ensure that the plan does not substantially discourage enrollment by specific patient populations, CMS will only approve specialty tiers under the following conditions:

- There is only one specialty tier exempt from cost-sharing exceptions.
- Cost-sharing is limited to 25% in the initial coverage range (or actuarially equivalent for plans with decreased or no deductible basic alternative design).
- Only plans with negotiated prices exceeding a threshold may be placed in the tier. The level is $500 a month in 2007 and $600 a month in 2008.

Formulary Changes During Plan Year

MMA provided that if plans removed drugs from their formularies during the year (or changed their preferred or tiered status), they were required to provide notice, on a timely basis, to CMS, affected enrollees, physicians, pharmacies and pharmacists. Observers expressed concerns about the implications of formulary changes on plan enrollees. In response, CMS emphasized that best practices call for limited changes during the plan year and outlined the following circumstances under which such changes can be made:

- Plans can expand formularies by adding drugs, lowering the tier of a drug (thereby reducing copayments or coinsurance), or deleting utilization management requirements.
- Plans cannot change therapeutic categories and classes during a year except to account for new therapeutic uses and newly approved Part D drugs.
- Plans can make formulary maintenace changes after March 1, such as replacing a brand name drug with a new generic drug or modifying formularies as a result of new information on safety or effectiveness. These changes require approval and 60 days notice to appropriate parties.

- Plans can only remove drugs from a formulary, move covered drugs to a less preferred tier status, or add utilization management requirements in accordance with approved procedures and after 60 days notice to appropriate parties. *Plans can make such changes only if enrollees currently taking the affected drugs are exempt from the formulary change for the remainder of the plan year.*

Plans are not required to obtain CMS approval or give 60 days notice when removing formulary drugs that have been withdrawn from the market by either the FDA or a product manufacturer.

Transition Policies

CMS has established transition standards intended to assure that new plan enrollees do not abruptly lose coverage for their drugs. Specifically, plans are required to provide a temporary supply fill anytime within the first 90 days of a beneficiary's enrollment in a plan. The supply must be for 30 days (unless the prescription is written for less than 30 days) for any nonformulary drug. The requirement also applies to drugs that are on a plan's formulary, but that require prior authorization or step therapy. In long-term care facilities, the transition policy provides for a 31-day fill, with multiple fills as necessary, during the first 90 days of a beneficiary's enrollment in a plan. After the 90-day period, the plan must provide a 31-day emergency supply while an exception is being processed. (CMS has specified 31 days because many long-term care pharmacies dispense medications in 31-day increments.) For contract year 2008, sponsors are required to ensure that the transition process information is prominently posted on their website.

CMS has noted that the purpose of the process is not just to provide a temporary fill of non-formulary drugs but rather to provide enrollees with sufficient time to work with their health care providers to switch to a therapeutically appropriate formulary alternative or to request an exception based on grounds of medical necessity.

Formulary Change Notice in Advance of Upcoming Year

As noted earlier, enrollees must receive an annual notice of change (ANOC) by October 31 prior to the next contract year. The upcoming year's formulary is viewed as a new formulary; therefore CMS does not require plans to identify specific drug changes impacting enrollees or require 60 days notice of change. However, enrollees have at least 60 days to review the new formulary and identify any changes.

CMS has outlined two options for providing a transition for enrollees whose drugs are no longer on the formulary. They may provide a transition process for current enrollees consistent with the transition process for new enrollees beginning January 1 of the new contract year. Alternatively, they can effectuate a transition for current enrollees prior to January 1. However, if plans have not successfully transitioned the affected enrollees to a therapeutically equivalent formulary alternative or processed an exceptions request by January 1, they are expected to provide a transition supply beginning January 1 until such time as they have effected a meaningful transition.

PHARMACY ACCESS

PDP sponsors are required to establish a pharmacy network sufficient to ensure access to covered Part D drugs for all enrollees. They must demonstrate that they provide (1) convenient access to retail pharmacies for all enrollees, (2) adequate access to home infusion pharmacies for all enrollees, (3) convenient access to long-term care (LTC) pharmacies for residents of LTC facilities, and (4) access to Indian Health Service, Tribes, or Urban Indian Programs (I/T/U) pharmacies operating in the sponsor's service area.

CMS can waive the standards in the case of (1) MA-PD plans that operate their own pharmacies, provided they can demonstrate convenient access, and (2) private-fee-for-service plans offering Part D coverage for drugs purchased from all pharmacies, provided they do not charge additional cost-sharing for drugs obtained from non-network pharmacies.

Retail Pharmacy Access

MMA defined convenient access to retail pharmacies as being no less favorable than those standards specified for the Department of Defense TRICARE regional pharmacy program as of March 13, 2003. The applicable Part D standards are as follows:

Plan Characteristics/Beneficiary Protections

- In urban areas, at least 90% of Medicare beneficiaries in the plan's service area, on average, live within 2 miles of a retail pharmacy participating in the plan's network.
- In suburban areas, at least 90% of Medicare beneficiaries in the plan's service area, on average, live within 5 miles of a retail pharmacy participating in the plan's network.
- In rural areas, at least 70% of Medicare beneficiaries in the plan's service area, on average, live within 15 miles of a retail pharmacy participating in the plan's network.

The inclusion of mail order pharmacies in Part D plan networks is optional. However, such plans do not count toward meeting the retail pharmacy access requirements. Plans that include mail order pharmacies in their networks must allow enrollees to receive benefits, such as extended (e.g., 90-day) supply of covered drugs through a network retail pharmacy. However, beneficiaries making this choice could be subject to higher cost sharing charges.

Part D sponsors may not restrict access to Part D drugs by limiting distribution through a subset of network pharmacies ("specialty pharmacies"), except when necessary to meet FDA limited distribution requirements or to ensure the appropriate dispensing of drugs that require extraordinary special handling, provider coordination, or patient education when such requirements cannot be met by a network pharmacy.

Long-Term Care (LTC) Pharmacy Access

Part D sponsors must offer standard LTC pharmacy network contracts to all LTC pharmacies operating in their service area that request such contracts. The pharmacy must be able to meet performance and service criteria specified by CMS as well as any standard terms and conditions established by the Part D sponsor for its network LTC pharmacies. Part D sponsors may not rely on out-of-network pharmacies to meet the LTC convenient access standards.

"Any Willing Pharmacy"

Part D sponsors are required to permit any pharmacy willing to accept the sponsor's standard contracting terms and conditions to participate in the plan's network. CMS notes that the sponsors standard terms and conditions may vary to accommodate geographic areas and types of pharmacies. However, all similarly situated pharmacies are to be offered the same standard terms and conditions.

A Part D pharmacy may not require a network pharmacy to accept insurance risk as a condition of participation in its pharmacy network.

PUBLIC DISCLOSURE OF PRICES

Part D sponsors are required to ensure that their network pharmacies inform enrollees of any price differential between a covered drug and the lowest price generic version of the drug that is therapeutically equivalent, bioequivalent, on the plan's formulary, and available at that pharmacy.

PRIVACY, CONFIDENTIALITY, AND ACCURACY OF ENROLLEE RECORDS

Plans must abide by all applicable federal and state laws regarding confidentiality and disclosure of any medical records that it maintains. Further, it must maintain the records in an accurate and timely manner and ensure timely access by enrollees to records and information pertaining to them.

GRIEVANCES, COVERAGE DETERMINATIONS, AND APPEALS

Part D plans are required to have procedures in place for handling grievances, for making timely coverage determinations, and for handling appeals of coverage determinations. They must ensure that all enrollees receive written information about these procedures.

Grievances

Grievances are complaints or disputes, other than those involving coverage determinations, expressing dissatisfaction with any aspect of the operations, activities, or behavior of a Part D plan, regardless of whether remedial action is requested. Grievances may include such things as complaints about the plan's customer service hours of operation, time to obtain a prescription, or pharmacy charges. A grievance may also include a complaint that the Part D plan refused to expedite a coverage determination or redetermination. A beneficiary with a grievance should file the complaint within 60 days of the event. The plan sponsor must respond on a timely basis.

Coverage Determinations

A coverage determination is any determination (either an approval or denial) made by the plan sponsor with regard to covered benefits. The following actions are considered coverage determinations:

- A decision about whether to provide or pay for a part D drug that the enrollee believes may be covered. This includes a decision not to pay because the drug is not on the plan's formulary, the drug is determined not medically necessary, or the drug is furnished by an out-of-network pharmacy.
- Failure to provide a coverage determination in a timely manner when a delay would adversely affect the health of the enrollee.
- A decision concerning a tiering exceptions request. MMA provided that if a Part D plan includes a tiered cost-sharing structure, a plan enrollee can request an exception to the structure. Under an exception, a nonpreferred drug could be covered as a preferred drug if the prescribing physician determined that the preferred drug for treatment of the same condition would not be as effective for the individual, would have adverse effects for the individual, or both.
- A decision concerning a formulary exceptions request. MMA provided that a beneficiary enrolled in a Part D plan can appeal a determination not to provide coverage for a drug not on the plan's formulary. The appeal can only be made if the prescribing physician determines that all covered Part D drugs on any tier of the formulary for treatment of the same condition would not be as

effective for the individual as the nonformulary drug, would have adverse effects for the individual, or both.
- A decision on the amount of cost-sharing.
- A decision whether the individual has, or has not, satisfied a prior authorization or other utilization management requirement.

A request for a coverage determination may be filed by the enrollee, the enrollee's appointed representative, or the enrollee's physician. The sponsor must notify the enrollee of its determinations within 72 hours of receipt of the request (or, in the case of an exceptions request, receipt of the physician's supporting statement). An enrollee can request an expedited decision; if the plan approves the request, it must make the determination within 24 hours.

Appeals

If the plan's coverage determination is unfavorable to the enrollee, it must provide the enrollee with a written denial notice that includes information on appeals rights. There are five levels of appeals.

Redetermination

The first level of appeal is a redetermination by the plan. An enrollee, or the appointed representative, may request a standard redetermination with respect to covered drug benefits or payments. An enrollee, the appointed representative or the enrollee's prescribing physician may request an expedited redetermination for covered drug benefits. The request should generally be filed within 60 days of the unfavorable coverage determination. The sponsor must provide the enrollee or prescribing physician with a reasonable opportunity to present evidence. Enrollees must be notified of the results within seven days in the case of standard redetermination. Enrollees requesting expedited redeterminations of a request for covered drugs must be notified of the results within 72 hours, if the plan accepts the expedited request.

The redetermination must be made by a person not involved in the original coverage determination. If the issue is the denial of coverage based on medical necessity, the redetermination must be made by a physician.

Reconsideration by an Independent Review Entity

An enrollee dissatisfied with a redetermination has a right to reconsideration by an independent review entity (IRE) that contracts with CMS for this purpose. Currently, MAXIMUS Federal Services is the Part D IRE.

An enrollee or an enrollee's appointed representative may request a standard or expedited reconsideration. The request must be made within 60 days of the redetermination. An enrollee's prescribing physician may not request a reconsideration on an enrollee's behalf unless the enrollee's physician is also the enrollee's appointed representative. The IRE must solicit the views of the prescribing physician. It is required to make a decision within seven days for a standard reconsideration and 72 hours for an expedited reconsideration.

Administrative Law Judge

The third level of appeal is an administrative law judge (ALJ). An enrollee or the appointed representative may request a hearing with an administrative law judge. An enrollee's prescribing physician may not request a hearing by an ALJ on an enrollee's behalf unless the enrollee's physician is also the enrollee's appointed representative. The request must be made within 60 days of the IRE decision letter. To get an ALJ hearing, the projected value of denied coverage must meet a minimum dollar amount ($110 in 2007). No time frames are specified for ALJ action.

Medicare Appeals Council

The fourth level of appeal is the Medicare Appeals Council (MAC). A beneficiary or the appointed representative may request a review by the MAC within 60 days of the ALJ decision. The MAC may grant or deny the request for review. If it grants the request, it may issue a final decision or dismissal, or remand the case to the ALJ with instructions on how to proceed with the case. No times frames are specified for a MAC review.

Federal District Court

The final appeal level is a Federal district court. A beneficiary or the appointed representative may request a review by a federal court within 60 days of the MAC decision notice. To receive a review by the court, the projected value of denied coverage must meet a minimum dollar amount ($1,130 in 2007).

COST CONTROL AND QUALITY IMPROVEMENT

Part D sponsors are required to have a drug utilization management program, quality assurance measures and systems, and a medication therapy management program.

Drug Utilization Management

Sponsors must establish a reasonable and appropriate drug utilization management program that (1) includes incentives to reduce costs when medically appropriate and (2) maintains policies and systems to assist in preventing over-utilization and under-utilization of prescribed medications.

Quality Assurance

The sponsor must have established quality assurance measures and systems to reduce medication errors and adverse drug interactions and improve medication use. Such measures and systems must provide that network providers are required to comply with state standards for pharmacy practice. They must also provide both for concurrent drug utilization review systems and retrospective review systems.

Medication Therapy Management

Each Part D Sponsor is required to incorporate a Medication Therapy Management Program (MTMP) into their plans' benefit structure. Each year, sponsors are required to submit a MTMP description to CMS for review and approval. A CMS-approved MTMP is one of several required elements in the development of sponsor' bids for the upcoming contract year.

An approved MTMP must (1) ensure optimum therapeutic outcomes for targeted beneficiaries through improved medication use; (2) reduce the risk of adverse events for targeted beneficiaries; (3) be developed in cooperation with licensed and practicing pharmacists and physicians; (4) be coordinated with any care management plan established for a targeted individual under a chronic care improvement program; (5) describe the resources and time required to implement the program if using outside personnel and establish the fees for pharmacists or others. The MTMP may be furnished by pharmacists or other qualified providers and may distinguish between services in ambulatory and institutional settings.

Targeted beneficiaries under a MTMP are enrollees who have chronic diseases, are taking multiple Part D drugs, and are likely to incur annual costs for covered drugs that exceed a level specified by the Secretary ($4,000 in 2007 and 2008).

CMS has outlined additional expectations for MTMPs. Beneficiaries enrolled in a MTMP cannot be disenrolled later in the year, even if they no longer meet one of the eligibility criteria. Plans will provide interventions for beneficiaries meeting all of the criteria regardless of the setting. The plan will not include discriminatory exclusion criteria.

E-PRESCRIBING

MMA required the development of electronic prescribing (e-prescribing) standards for the Part D program. The first (or "foundation") e-prescribing standards, which became effective in 2006, created uniform system requirements for several e-prescribing functions, such as eligibility and benefits queries between prescribers and Part D sponsors. In accordance with the MMA, CMS also conducted a pilot study to assess the feasibility of creating additional e-prescribing standards. On November 17, 2007, CMS issued a notice of proposed rule-making to adopt standards for transactions related to formulary and benefit information and medication history.

Providers and pharmacies are not required to use e-prescribing; however, a provider or pharmacy that does e-prescribe for Part D beneficiaries is required to comply with any applicable final standards that are in effect. Further, all Part D plans are required to maintain e-prescribing systems that conform to the final standards.

PAYMENTS TO PLANS

CMS makes four types of payments to Part D plans: (1) direct subsidy payments, (2) reinsurance payments, (3) low-income subsidy payments, and (4) risk-sharing payments.

DIRECT SUBSIDIES

Medicare makes per capita monthly payments to plans for each Part D enrollee. The payment is equal to the plan's approved standardized bid amount, adjusted by the plan beneficiaries' health status and risk, and reduced by the base beneficiary premium for the plan.

Plan Bid

As noted earlier, plans are required to submit, not later than the first Monday in June, a bid for the following year. The bid is to include an estimate of its average monthly revenue requirements to provide qualified prescription drug benefits (including any supplemental coverage) for a Part D eligible individual with a national average risk profile. The bid includes costs (including administrative costs and return on investment/profit) for which the plan is responsible. The bid is to exclude costs paid by enrollees, payments expected to be made by CMS for reinsurance and any other costs for which the sponsor is not responsible. CMS reviews the bids, negotiates with plans, and approves the bids.

National Average Monthly Bid Amount

CMS then computes a *national average monthly bid amount* from approved bids. This is to be a weighted average of the standardized bid amount for each prescription drug plan. For PDPs, the standardized bid amount is that portion of a plan's bid attributable to basic prescription drug coverage; for MA-PDs , it is the portion of the accepted bid that is attributable to basic prescription drug coverage.

In calculating the nationwide average, CMS is to weight each plan's bid by its share of total enrollment. In 2006, the first year of Part D, there was no prior PDP enrollment information; therefore each PDP plan was weighted equally (though MA-PD bids were enrollment weighted if they had 2005 MA enrollment). Rather than immediately moving to full enrollment weighting in 2007, CMS provided for a phase-in under its demonstration authority ("Medicare Demonstration to Limit Annual Changes in Part D Premiums Due to Beneficiary Choice of Low-Cost Plans"). In 2007, 80% of the national monthly bid amount was based on the 2006 averaging methodology and 20% on the enrollment weighted average. In 2008, 40% is based on the 2006 averaging methodology and 60% on the enrollment weighted average. CMS chose this phase-in approach because with 2006 enrollment heavily weighted toward lower cost plans, immediate use of the enrollment weighting methodology would have resulted in lower direct subsidies, and by extension higher beneficiary premiums.

The calculation of the national average monthly bid amount does not include bids submitted by MSA plans, MA private fee-for-service plans, specialized MA plans for special needs populations, PACE programs and plans established through reasonable cost contracts.

The national average monthly bid amount for 2007 is $80.43; it is $80.52 in 2008.

Payment to Plans

Individual plan bids are adjusted for expected case mix. This adjustment takes into account variation in costs among plans for basic coverage based on the differences in actuarial risk of different enrollees being served. Per capita monthly direct subsidy payments equal this adjusted amount minus the base beneficiary premium. (See discussion below for how beneficiary premiums are calculated.)

REINSURANCE SUBSIDIES

As noted in the discussion of prescription drug benefits, Part D plans pay all drug costs above the catastrophic threshold ($5,451.25 in 2007, $5,726.25 in 2008) except for nominal beneficiary cost-sharing.

Medicare subsidizes 80% of the plans' costs for catastrophic coverage. CMS makes reinsurance subsidy payments to plans in behalf of those individuals who have actually incurred such costs. Payments are made on a monthly basis during the year based on either estimated or incurred costs, with final reconciliation made after the close of the year.

In the case of private fee-for-service plans offering drug coverage, CMS determines reinsurance payments by basing the amount on CMS' estimate of the amount that would be paid if it were a coordinated care plan and takes into account average payments for populations of similar risk in such plans.

RISK CORRIDOR PAYMENTS

MMA established risk corridors which were intended to limit a plan's overall risks or profits under the new program. By using risk corridors, Medicare is able to limit a plan's potential losses by financing some of the higher than expected costs. Similarly, Medicare is able to limit a plan's potential gains by recouping excessive costs. Over time, as more experience is gained with the program, the risk corridors are widened, thereby increasing the insurance risk borne by the plans. The risk corridor provisions do not apply to private fee-for-service plans.

Risk corridors are defined as specified percentages above and below a target amount. The target amount is defined as total payments paid to the plan, taking into account the amount paid by the CMS and enrollees, based on the standardized bid amount, risk adjusted, and reduced by total administrative expenses assumed in the bid. No payment adjustments are made if adjusted allowable costs for the plan are at least equal to the first threshold lower limit of the first risk corridor but not greater than the first threshold upper limit of the risk corridor for the year (i.e., if the plans are within the first risk corridor). A portion of any plan spending above or below these levels is subject to risk adjustment. If adjusted allowable costs exceed the first threshold upper limit, then payments are increased. If adjusted allowable costs are below the first threshold lower limit, then payments are reduced. Adjusted allowable costs are reduced by reinsurance and subsidy payments. (See **Table 3**.)

During 2006 and 2007, plans are at full risk for adjusted allowable risk corridor costs between 2.5% below and 2.5% above the target. Plans with adjusted allowable costs above this level receive increased payments. If their costs are between 2.5% of the target (first threshold upper limit) and 5% of the target (second threshold upper limit), they are at risk for 25% of the increased amount; that is, their payments equal 75% of adjusted allowable costs for spending in this range. If their costs are above 5% of the target they are at risk for 25% of the costs between the first and second threshold upper limits and 20% of the costs above that amount. That is, their payments equal 80% of the adjusted allowable costs over the second threshold upper limit. Conversely, if plans fall below the target, they share the savings with the government. They have to refund 75% of the savings if costs fall between 2.5% and 5% below the target level, and 80% of any amounts below 5% of the target.

For 2008-2011, the risk corridors are modified. Plans are at full risk for drug spending between 5.0% below and 5% above the target level. Plans are at risk for 50% of spending exceeding 5.0% and below 10.0% of the target level. Additionally, they are at risk for 20% of any spending exceeding 10% of the target level. Conversely, if plans fall below the target, they have to refund 50% of the savings if costs fall between 5% and 10% below the target level and 80% of any amounts below 10% of the target. Beginning in 2012, CMS may increase the target levels above the 5% and 10% levels.

Table 3. Plan Liability Under Risk Corridor Provisions

Risk Corridor	Plan Liability for Costs Above and Below Target
2006-2007	
Costs below 95% of the target	80% refund
Costs between 95% and 97.5% of the target	75% refund
Costs between 97.5% and 102.5% of the target	Full risk
Costs between 102.5% and 105% of the target	Risk for 25% of amount
Costs over 105% of the target	Risk for 20% of amount
2008-2011	
Costs below 90% of the target	80% refund
Costs between 90% and 95% of the target	50% refund
Costs between 95% and 105 % of the target	Full risk
Costs between 105 % and 110 % of the target	Risk for 50% of amount
Costs over 110% of the target	Risk for 20% of amount

LOW-INCOME SUBSIDY (LIS) PAYMENTS

CMS makes additional payments to plans on behalf of persons entitled to low-income subsidies. These payments are for premium and cost-sharing charges which would otherwise be paid by the beneficiary except for the fact that they are entitled to subsidies. (See "Low-Income Individuals" section below).

RECONCILIATION

CMS makes prospective payments to plans based on their bids. Following the close of the calendar year, CMS makes retroactive adjustments to reflect actual plan experience. Prospective payments for reinsurance and low-income subsidy payments are compared to actual incurred costs and other related data, and appropriate adjustments are made to the plan payments. The calculation is based on costs actually incurred and must be net of any direct or indirect remuneration (including discounts, chargebacks or rebates). Direct subsidy payments to the plans are adjusted to reflect updated data about beneficiary health status and enrollment. In addition, any necessary adjustments are made to reflect risk sharing under the risk corridor provisions.

In October 2007, CMS announced that it would collect $4 billion from Part D drug plan sponsors due to lower-than-expected drug costs in 2006. It stated that it would be collecting these funds from plans due to the fact that actual drug costs for almost all Part D plans were below expected levels in their 2006 bids. It cited several factors leading to lower spending, including the fact that 2006 marked the first time that plans were bidding on the new Part D program and the fact there were higher levels of generic drug utilization in Part D than had been anticipated. It further noted that plans submitted their bids for the 2006 contracting year in June 2005. The 2006 bids were therefore somewhat uncertain predictions of what would actually happen when the drug benefit began in 2006. CMS expects that as experience with Part D grows, plan bid submissions will more closely reflect actual costs. It stated that the 2007 bid submissions were significantly lower than those submitted in 2006 and were a reflection of the actual 2006 Part D drug program experience. Therefore, CMS anticipates that amounts collected from or paid to plans in future years as a result of final reconciliation and risk adjustment will be lower than that for the 2006 plan year.[6]

BENEFICIARY PREMIUMS

Beneficiaries pay monthly premiums for Part D coverage. Payments vary by the plan selected. On average, beneficiary premiums are to represent roughly 25.5% of the cost of basic coverage.

The monthly premium is uniform for all persons enrolled in the plan (except for those receiving low-income subsidies or those subject to a late enrollment penalty). It equals the base beneficiary premium, as adjusted to reflect the difference between the plan's standardized bid amount and the nationwide average bid.

PREMIUM CALCULATION

Base Beneficiary Premium

The base beneficiary premium for a Part D plan equals the product of the beneficiary premium percentage and the national average monthly bid amount (see calculation under "Direct Subsidies," above). The beneficiary premium percentage is equal to 25.5%, divided by 100% minus a percentage equal to total reinsurance payments divided by the sum of such reinsurance payments and total payments the Secretary estimates will be paid to prescription drug plans in a year that are attributable to the standardized bid amount (taking into account amounts paid by CMS and enrollees).

The base beneficiary monthly premium is $27.35 in 2007 and $27.93 in 2008.

Adjustments

Once the base beneficiary premium is calculated, it is adjusted up or down, as appropriate, to reflect any difference between the plan's standardized bid amount and the nationwide average bid amount. Thus, beneficiaries in plans with higher costs for standard coverage face higher than average premiums for such coverage, while enrollees in lower cost plans pay lower than average premiums for such coverage.

Premiums are further increased to reflect any supplemental benefits or any late enrollment penalty and decreased if the individual is entitled to a low-income subsidy. Additionally, enrollees in MA-PD plans may see a decrease if plans use rebates, based on Parts A and B benefit costs, to buy down the Part D premium.

PROGRAM FINANCING

Medicare Part D is financed through a combination of Federal general revenues, beneficiary premiums, and state contributions. Revenues are credited to a separate account, the Medicare Prescription Drug Account, in the Medicare Part B trust fund.

GENERAL REVENUES AND BENEFICIARY PREMIUMS

General Revenues

General revenues are transferred from the Treasury to the Part D Account on an as-needed basis to support the portion of program expenditures funded by federal subsidies.

Beneficiary Premiums

Beneficiaries may have their premiums deducted from their social security or other federal benefit payments; these are then forwarded to Part D plans on their behalf. Alternatively, they can pay their premiums directly to the Part D plan. Both types of payments are shown in the statement of the Part D account in the annual Medicare trustees report.

STATE CONTRIBUTIONS

Effective January 1, 2006, states are no longer providing coverage for Part D drugs for their dual eligible population under Medicaid. They could be expected to see a reduction in their Medicaid spending as a result of this transfer. However, MMA contained a provision (labeled by some as the "clawback provision") that requires states to continue to assume a portion of these costs. The formula specified in law is based on a proxy for what states would otherwise be spending on drugs for the dual eligibles in the absence of MMA. In 2006, states assumed 90% of these costs; over the next nine years the states' contribution phases-down to 75% in 2015.

Formula for State Contribution Amount

States are required to pay the Secretary each month an amount equal to the *product* of the following three factors:

- The projected monthly per capita drug payment which is product of: base year (2003) state Medicaid per capita expenditures for covered Part D drugs for full benefit dual eligible persons (reduced by any rebates received) and the current state matching rate. This amount is increased each year (beginning in 2004) by the applicable growth factor; beginning in 2007 this is the per capita percentage increase in Part D expenditures.
- Total number of full benefit dual eligibles for the state for the month.
- The applicable percentage factor (90% in 2006, 88 1/3% in 2007, 86 2/3 % in 2008, decreased each year by 1 2/3 percentage points until 2015 and later when it is 75%).

Impact on States

A review for the National Association of State Medicaid Directors found that most states report that the combination of the transition of dual eligibles to Part D coupled with state clawback payments have not resulted in significant state savings. Only 10 states reported paying less in 2007 for dual eligibles than when the state provided drugs directly to this population. Further, most states have not implemented wrap-around coverage for Part D cost-sharing amounts for low-income subsidy beneficiaries.[7]

PART D ACCOUNT DATA

MMA created a separate Part D account within the Medicare Part B trust fund. The 2007 Medicare Trustees Report stated that in calendar year 2006, total Part D revenues were $48.1 billion. This included $3.5 billion in beneficiary premiums, $39.1 billion in government contributions, $5.5 billion in state contributions and $13 million interest on investments. Total Part D benefits (including employer subsidy payments) were $47.3 billion with an additional $0.3 billion for federal administrative expenses. (See **Table 4.**)

Table 4. Statement of Operations of Part D Account, Calendar Year 2006 (in millions)

Total Assets at Beginning of Year	$0
Revenues	**$48,070.2**
Premiums from Enrollees	$3,450.3
Premiums deducted from social security checks	$1,184.8
Premiums paid directly to plans	$2,265.5
Government Contributions	39,133.1
Prescription drug benefits	38,825.9
Administrative expenses	307.2
Payments from States	5,474.2
Interest on Investments	12.6
Expenditures	**$47,276.3**
Benefit Payments	46,969.1
Federal Administrative Expenses	307.2
Assets of fund at End of Year	**$793.9**

Source: 2007 Annual Report of the Boards of Trustees of the Federal Hospital Insurance and Federal Supplementary Insurance Trust Funds.

The trustees reported that the 2006 expenditures were less than had been predicted in the 2005 and 2006 trustees report. They attributed this change to several factors including a slowdown in the growth in prescription drug spending; the fact that savings from retail discounts, manufacturer rebates, and utilization management were achieved in 2006 rather than over several years as had been previously assumed; and the fact that significantly fewer beneficiaries joined the program than initially anticipated and that some who joined enrolled after the beginning of the year.

Employer Subsidies

MMA included provisions designed to encourage employers to continue to offer drug benefits to their Medicare-eligible retirees. It provided a subsidy for a portion of retiree drug costs and exempted these subsidy payments from federal taxes.

Qualifications

Qualified Plans

CMS makes the subsidy payments to employers or unions offering qualified retiree prescription drug coverage. Qualified plans are defined as those offering drug benefits at least actuarially equivalent to "standard coverage."

Qualifying Covered Retiree

Subsidy payments are made on behalf of an individual covered under the retiree health plan who is entitled to enroll under a PDP or MA-PD plan but elects not to. Subsidies are linked to an individual's status as a retired participant in the qualified group health plan or as the Medicare-enrolled spouse or dependent of the retired participant. Thus, a sponsor offering qualified coverage for dependants will be able to claim coverage for a Part D eligible dependent of a retired participant, even if the retiree is under age 65 and not Part D eligible. However, the sponsor will not be able to claim coverage for a Part D eligible dependent of an active employee.

An individual retiree can elect to enroll in Part D, even if the former employer has elected to take the subsidy. However, this decision may have consequences. It is possible the individual could lose employer-sponsored drug coverage or both employer-sponsored medical and drug coverage. Further, any payments made by the employer plan would not count toward meeting the true out-of-pocket (TROOP) requirements (See earlier discussion of Part D benefits.)

SUBSIDY BENEFITS

Subsidy payments equal 28% of a retiree's gross drug costs between specified levels ($265-$5,350 in 2007; $275-$5,600 in 2008). The dollar amounts are adjusted annually by the percentage increase in Medicare per capita prescription drug costs.) Subsidy payments to employers and unions are not subject to federal tax.

ALTERNATIVES

Employers or unions may select an alternative option (instead of taking the subsidy) with respect to Part D. They may elect to pay a portion of the Part D premiums. They may also elect to provide enhanced coverage that may be provided through supplementary or "wrap around" benefits. This approach may have some financial consequences for the employer or union since third party payments do not count toward TROOP. Thus, if an employer chooses to pay some of the Part D cost-sharing on behalf of its retirees, this would have the effect of delaying the point at which the Part D catastrophic coverage would begin. The employer could therefore end up paying some costs which would otherwise be covered under the catastrophic portion of the Part D benefit.

Employers or unions may also contract with a PDP or MA-PD to offer the coverage. Finally, they may become a Part D plan sponsor themselves for their retirees.

SUBSIDY DATA

Employer Actions

A December 2006 survey by Kaiser Family Foundation and Hewitt[8] noted that its survey of 302 large private-sector firms with 1,000 or more employees showed that the majority of plan sponsors (78%) would seek the subsidy in 2007 (compared with 82% in 2006). Six percent said they were likely to supplement the benefit; another 6% said they intended to contract with a PDP or MA-PD to offer additional coverage, and 2% said they intended to become a PDP. Eight percent said they were likely to discontinue prescription drug coverage.

Retirees Covered

In January 2007, the Secretary of HHS announced that 6.9 million persons were in retiree plans receiving a subsidy. An estimated 100 thousand were in plans with coverage at least as good as Medicare's but without a subsidy. Further, an estimated 3.3 million beneficiaries were in TRICARE and the Federal Employees Health Benefits program (FEHB); the federal government elected not to take the employer subsidy for these individuals on the grounds that it would be merely subsidizing itself.

ISSUES

As of January 2008, Part D began its third year of operation. While early startup issues have generally been resolved, some issues remain. The following highlights a few of these.

LOW-INCOME INDIVIDUALS

A major focus of Part D is the enhanced coverage provided to low-income individuals through the low-income subsidy (LIS) program. Despite extensive federal, state, and local outreach efforts, not all persons potentially eligible have enrolled in the program. As of January 2007, CMS estimated that 3.3 million persons eligible for LIS had neither signed up for Part D nor had coverage through another source. It is not immediately clear why some individuals have failed to enroll, though several factors, including a lack of program awareness and the nature of the application process itself play a role. The assets limitations are viewed by some as being too low, thereby precluding otherwise eligible persons from gaining coverage.

A second issue of concern to the low-income population is the large number of persons required to change plans each year because the premium for their current plan no longer falls below the low-income subsidy level. Some observers have suggested that when making the low-income subsidy calculation (see earlier discussion) the MA-PD enrollment should be removed from the calculation. Their inclusion in the calculation has the effect of lowering the benchmark, thereby forcing a higher number of persons enrolled in PDPs to change plans if they are to remain in zero premium plans.

HIGH-INCOME ENROLLEES

On average, beneficiary premiums account for 25.5% of expected total Part D costs for basic coverage; federal general revenues account for most of the remaining costs. Some persons have suggested that higher income persons should pay a higher percentage of their costs. Except for persons entitled to low-income subsidies, all persons selecting a particular Part D plan pay the same monthly premium amount.

The President's FY2008 Budget proposal would establish income-related premiums for Part D. Though specifics were not provided, it was expected that the percentage increases would be tied to the benchmark premium amount for basic coverage. Under the proposal, the income thresholds would be the same as those currently established for income-relating Part B premiums and therefore affect the same people. Further, as proposed for Part B, the income thresholds would not be updated in future years. Consequently, each year the number of beneficiaries subject to the higher premium would increase. The budget included estimated savings of $357 million in FY2008 and $3.242 billion over the five-year budget period.

At the time the proposal was presented, CMS estimated that it would affect 4.3% of beneficiaries in 2008, rising to 6.7% of beneficiaries in 2017. This is a slightly smaller percentage affected by the Part D proposal than by the Part B proposal. This reflects the fact that many high-income enrollees have alternative sources of prescription drug coverage, such as through coverage provided by former employers.

Some observers (who had also opposed income-relating the Part B premium) suggest that this approach would further move Medicare from its entitlement nature.

BENEFICIARY EXPERIENCE

When MMA was enacted, few observers expected beneficiaries to have a choice among so many drug plans. Some argue that the large number of plans available to beneficiaries may complicate their choices. Given that enrollment tends to be heavily concentrated in plans offered by a limited number of sponsors, it is likely that the number of available options will decline over time.

Beneficiaries have tended to enroll in plans with low premiums, and zero or low deductibles. However, in the absence of concrete data, it is not clear whether this is always the best choice for the beneficiary.

Most Part D enrollees did not change plan enrollment from 2006 to 2007. As noted in the "key facts section" below, premiums for the most popular plans are rising in 2008; plan sponsors may also make other changes including changing copayments or utilization controls for particular drugs. Despite the fact that plans are required to notify beneficiaries of changes, it is not clear how many are aware of the year-to-year modifications. It is also not clear whether beneficiaries will modify their plan choices.

At this point, information is not available to assess the impact of Part D over time on changes in drug utilization patterns and out-of-pocket costs.

DRUG PRICES

Noninterference Clause

Some observers have recommended striking the noninterference provision in the law. They claim that permitting CMS to be involved in negotiating drug prices would result in additional savings. Other observers state that plans are already achieving price reductions. The Congressional Budget Office has stated that removal of the noninterference clause would be unlikely to achieve significant additional savings, particularly if CMS were not allowed to establish a formulary or use other tools to reduce prices.[9]

Data

A considerable amount of plan-specific data is available on the WEB. However, certain information (for example, information dealing with price trends or price concessions such as rebates) is proprietary. The gaps in data make it difficult to provide a complete picture of the program's impact. The Government Accountability Office (GAO) was recently denied access to some Part D data. CMS has stated that MMA prohibits disclosure to other agencies.

PHARMACIES

Pharmacies are not required to process claims within a specified time period. Thirty days is considered the standard, though some pharmacies, particularly those located in rural areas allege that some claims take up to 45 days. They state that claims should be paid within 14 days. Some observers state that some pharmacies, particularly small pharmacies, are unable to handle the lag and are being driven out of business.

KEY PART D FACTS

ENROLLMENT

Enrollment by State

The annual open enrollment period for 2007 closed December 31, 2006. As of January 2007, approximately 23.9 million Medicare beneficiaries were enrolled in PDP and MA-PD plans. An additional 6.9 million beneficiaries had prescription drug coverage through a former employer that is receiving a federal subsidy for a portion of such coverage. Approximately 8.2 million beneficiaries had drug coverage through another source including persons with Federal Employees Health Benefits (FEHB) coverage and TRICARE coverage. An estimated 4.1 million or 10% of Medicare beneficiaries had no drug coverage. **Table 5** shows the nationwide distribution of Medicare enrollees by the source of drug coverage.

Table 5. Total Number of Medicare Beneficiaries with Drug Coverage, as of January 16, 2007
(in millions)

Coverage from Medicare or a Former Employer	34.17
Coverage from Medicare	*23.90*
Stand-Alone PDP	10.98
MA	6.65
Dual Eligible Automatically Enrolled	6.27
Coverage from Former Employer	*10.27*
Retiree Drug Subsidy (RDS)	6.94
FEHB Retiree Coverage	1.47
TRICARE Retiree Coverage	1.86
Additional Sources of Coverage	**4.86**
Veterans Affairs	1.85
Indian Health service	.03
Active Workers with Medicare Secondary Payer	2.57
Other Retiree Coverage, not RDS	0.10
State Pharmaceutical Assistance Programs	0.31
TOTAL	**39.03**

Source: CMS, January 30, 2007.
Note: An estimated 4.1 million persons or 10% of beneficiaries had no drug coverage.

Table 6 shows the state-by-state distribution of the 34.17 million persons (shown in Table 5) with drug coverage through Part D or a former employer receiving the employer subsidy. The table also shows the state-by-state distribution of the approximately 9.1 million enrollees who were receiving low-income subsidy assistance. An additional 3.3 million persons were thought to be eligible for such assistance, but were not enrolled.

Table 6. Beneficiaries with Coverage Through Medicare or a Former Employer and Low-Income Subsidy Recipients, by State, as of January 16, 2007

State	Total Medicare Beneficiaries	Beneficiaries with Creditable Drug Coverage	Beneficiaries in Stand-Alone PDPs	Beneficiaries in Medicare Advantage Drug Plans (MA-PDs)	Dual Eligibles (Auto-Enrolled into PDPs)	Beneficiaries in Employer Plans Taking Retiree Drug Subsidies	Federal Retirees (Tricare, FEHB)	Estimated Number with Unknown Creditable Drug Coverage Status	LIS Beneficiaries
United States	43,404,884	34,167,178	10,976,906	6,654,373	6,270,154	6,937,852	3,327,893	8,872,572	9,181,180
Alabama	765,173	641,979	233,166	89,753	104,362	124,236	90,462	123,194	221,700
Alaska	53,218	42,693	9,880	167	11,926	12,456	8,264	10,525	13,870
Arizona	797,108	666,514	146,832	262,697	69,461	104,335	83,189	130,594	144,870
Arkansas	479,834	379,849	185,540	23,575	73,611	52,625	44,498	99,985	132,710
California	4,325,861	3,635,081	623,751	1,321,828	940,312	427,286	321,904	690,780	1,120,060
Colorado	529,442	448,930	113,831	144,271	47,378	76,699	66,751	80,512	88,680
Connecticut	537,386	409,655	163,407	41,871	70,106	113,599	20,672	127,731	98,470
Delaware	128,690	107,425	50,564	1,293	11,397	32,769	11,402	21,265	24,020
District of Columbia	77,128	57,721	11,398	5,148	16,197	3,956	21,022	19,407	20,210
Florida	3,094,899	2,485,285	652,990	685,760	385,277	473,079	288,179	609,614	571,600
Georgia	1,045,818	862,107	383,777	64,377	164,680	133,977	115,296	183,711	288,620
Guam	NA	NA	NA	NA	NA	NA	NA	NA	NA
Hawaii	186,157	160,867	38,186	56,515	25,204	8,315	32,647	25,290	34,670
Idaho	193,207	148,714	66,452	21,846	20,818	20,432	19,166	44,493	34,480
Illinois	1,734,572	1,343,089	569,312	89,356	263,160	353,439	67,822	391,483	324,250
Indiana	922,883	709,213	324,733	29,955	109,306	203,038	42,181	213,670	165,260
Iowa	499,314	397,416	230,178	27,809	59,667	55,352	24,410	101,898	82,170
Kansas	408,800	305,737	173,769	22,168	43,046	31,876	34,878	103,063	67,160

Table 6. Continued

State	Total Medicare Beneficiaries	Beneficiaries with Creditable Drug Coverage	Beneficiaries in Stand-Alone PDPs	Beneficiaries in Medicare Advantage Drug Plans (MA-PDs)	Dual Eligibles (Auto-Enrolled into PDPs)	Beneficiaries in Employer Plans Taking Retiree Drug Subsidies	Federal Retirees (Tricare, FEHB)	Estimated Number with Unknown Creditable Drug Coverage Status	LIS Beneficiaries
Kentucky	690,918	545,604	239,065	37,915	98,502	127,373	42,749	145,314	190,560
Louisiana	659,249	498,541	151,222	85,154	124,943	93,869	43,353	160,708	183,000
Maine	239,424	183,520	82,696	2,104	48,524	29,039	21,157	55,904	66,930
Maryland	708,981	560,681	192,427	33,989	64,962	147,936	121,367	148,300	120,560
Massachusetts	999,121	776,727	191,215	143,390	195,656	193,802	52,664	222,394	238,690
Michigan	1,519,223	1,207,073	305,782	178,355	204,412	472,574	45,950	312,150	266,590
Minnesota	711,498	574,786	242,602	147,642	72,542	78,221	33,779	136,712	123,180
Mississippi	465,962	365,066	150,134	10,350	131,388	30,577	42,617	100,896	161,530
Missouri	930,083	742,130	266,650	130,437	152,983	124,398	67,662	187,953	192,750
Montana	150,764	114,784	58,991	9,798	16,473	15,061	14,461	35,980	24,970
Nebraska	266,386	213,837	118,690	16,240	33,096	25,595	20,216	52,549	43,950
Nevada	302,537	242,979	55,422	88,748	23,438	41,049	34,322	59,558	44,900
New Hampshire	190,271	135,414	59,265	2,036	21,211	35,789	17,113	54,857	30,860
New Jersey	1,261,180	970,604	384,718	93,488	143,992	287,847	60,559	290,576	223,600
New Mexico	270,105	226,800	59,229	54,089	38,967	39,921	34,594	43,305	64,550
New York	2,858,747	2,073,158	375,098	481,196	547,469	576,824	92,571	785,589	688,800
North Carolina	1,288,827	1,067,585	396,945	124,516	231,549	206,359	108,216	221,242	339,190
North Dakota	105,800	84,815	58,261	2,932	11,543	4,997	7,082	20,985	17,590
Ohio	1,797,320	1,444,753	375,261	260,227	202,382	525,005	81,878	352,567	314,370
Oklahoma	550,500	435,411	187,259	49,185	80,194	53,014	65,759	115,089	120,280

Table 6. Continued

State	Total Medicare Beneficiaries	Beneficiaries with Creditable Drug Coverage	Beneficiaries in Stand-Alone PDPs	Beneficiaries in Medicare Advantage Drug Plans (MA-PDs)	Dual Eligibles (Auto-Enrolled into PDPs)	Beneficiaries in Employer Plans Taking Retiree Drug Subsidies	Federal Retirees (Tricare, FEHB)	Estimated Number with Unknown Creditable Drug Coverage Status	LIS Beneficiaries
Oregon	546,754	432,091	164,169	131,292	45,691	46,769	44,170	114,663	93,260
Pennsylvania	2,174,756	1,692,994	521,340	555,023	174,160	327,632	114,839	481,762	380,470
Puerto Rico	611,993	402,871	45,909	329,783	3,379	12,105	11,695	209,122	4,750
Residence Unknown	NA	41,076	4,982	2,161	2,174	NA	31,759	NA	NA
Rhode Island	176,960	138,560	31,522	53,907	27,456	12,655	13,020	38,400	40,660
South Carolina	654,600	542,680	187,009	37,631	122,997	119,731	75,312	111,920	169,930
South Dakota	127,175	101,037	64,536	5,322	13,164	6,661	11,354	26,138	21,960
Tennessee	933,031	772,236	235,118	117,599	225,655	123,417	70,447	160,795	278,670
Texas	2,570,082	2,132,859	780,684	297,847	363,889	423,086	267,353	437,223	666,120
Utah	237,900	193,395	72,082	31,775	22,895	32,427	34,216	44,505	32,830
Vermont	98,336	77,607	35,910	298	17,097	18,130	6,172	20,729	25,740
Virgin Islands	NA	7,414	3,793	68	40	3,274	239	NA	100
Virginia	1,002,150	806,145	327,334	56,264	116,170	122,003	184,374	196,005	198,160
Washington	831,236	647,097	232,162	92,584	105,586	115,166	101,599	184,139	145,820
West Virginia	363,200	287,117	115,004	15,637	48,984	87,657	19,835	76,083	85,820
Wisconsin	844,212	571,231	195,557	85,042	114,419	142,641	33,572	272,981	136,400
Wyoming	72,489	54,225	31,097	1,960	6,264	7,779	7,125	18,264	10,870

Source: The Henry J. Kaiser Family Foundation, State health facts, Medicare Beneficiaries with Creditable Prescription Drug Coverage by Type, as of January 16, 2007, and Medicare Drug Benefit Enrollees with the Low-Income Subsidy, as of 1/16/07.

Note: Number With Unknown creditable drug coverage status include 4.86 million with creditable coverage.

Plan Enrollment[10]

Part D enrollment is highly concentrated. In 2007, two organizations, UHC-PacifiCare and Humana, captured more than 40% of all Part D enrollees. These two organizations had the largest number and share of Part D enrollees in both stand-alone PDPs and MA-PDs. The top four organizations (including Wellpoint, Inc. and Member Health Inc.) captured 54% of enrollment. The top 10 organizations captured 72%. All of the top 10 organizations offered multiple plans and all but Kaiser Permanente offered both stand alone PDP and MA-PD plans.

In 2007, thirteen percent of Part D enrollees were in AARP's Medicare Rx Plan (offered by UHC-PacifiCare). This figure actually represented a decline from 2006, possibly because some persons shifted to a lower premium AARP offering, the AARP Medicare Savers Plan, which was also one of the top ten plans, in terms of enrollment.

Humana sponsored three of the top ten plans in 2007. The two PDP offerings, in second and third place, captured 9% and 5% of the market. Enrollment in its private fee-for-service plan increased significantly from 2006, due to a dramatic increase in market offerings.

Plan Features[11]

In 2007, only 14% of enrollees were in plans offering the defined standard Part D benefit. Half (51%) were enrolled in plans that offered actuarially equivalent benefits, while 35% were in plans that provided an enhanced benefit. Over three-quarters (79%) of enrollees in MA-PD plans had enhanced benefits, while only 21% of PDP enrollees had such coverage. Over half of PDP enrollees were in plans with no deductible while almost all of MA-PD enrollees had no deductible.

In 2007, 85% of enrollees were in plans with no gap coverage; 12% had coverage for some generics in the gap, and 3% had coverage for both brand name and generic drugs in the gap. Eight of the top ten plans offering both generic and brand coverage in the gap were MA-PD plans. One PDP (SierraRxPlus PDP) offering full gap coverage in 2007 is not offering such coverage in 2008.

It should be noted that low-income enrollees receiving LIS assistance have partial or full subsidized coverage in the gap. This group represents close to 40% of enrollees. When both those with LIS assistance and some gap coverage are taken into account, approximately half of enrollees (49%) of enrollees had no gap coverage in 2007.

2008 PLAN OVERVIEW

Table 7 provides an overview of PDP plan offerings for 2008. The number of plan offerings ranges from 47 in Alaska to 63 in West Virginia and Pennsylvania. The number of plans with premiums below the low income benchmark or with gap coverage is significantly lower.

Table 7 shows a wide range in premiums for PDP plans. Plans with higher premiums typically offer broader coverage. It should be noted that while the essentially the same plan may be offered in a number of PDP regions (or nationwide) the premiums for the plan are not likely to be the same in all PDP regions.

Table 7. Stand-Alone PDPs: Characteristics by State, 2008

State	Number of Plans	Number Below Low-Income Benchmark	Some Gap Coverage[a]	Monthly Premium	
				Low	High
Alabama	53	15	15	$18.00	$98.00
Alaska	47	15	14	$14.70	$99.50
Arizona	51	7	15	$9.80	$99.50
Arkansas	55	18	16.	$13.00	$98.00
California	56	9	15	$14.30	$102.70
Colorado	55	12	16	$15.60	$99.50
Connecticut	51	14	15	$14.60	$99.50
Delaware	52	18	15	$16.10	$97.50
District of Columbia	52	18	15	$16.10	$97.50
Florida	58	8	18	$12.10	$97.50
Georgia	54	18	15	$16.60	$97.50
Hawaii	49	10	15	$13.70	$99.50
Idaho	54	14	15	$17.10	$99.50
Illinois	53	19	15	$17.70	$97.50
Indiana	52	17	15	$17.30	$98.00
Iowa	52	16	16	$13.90	$99.00
Kansas	52	17	15	$14.90	$99.50
Kentucky	52	17	15	$17.30	$98.00
Louisiana	50	10	14	$14.30	$97.50

Table 7. Continued

State	Number of Plans	Number Below Low-Income Benchmark	Some Gap Coverage[a]	Monthly Premium Low	Monthly Premium High
Maine	53	18	16	$14.80	$99.50
Maryland	52	18	15	$16.10	$97.50
Massachusetts	51	14	15	$14.60	$99.50
Michigan	55	17	16	$17.90	$97.50
Minnesota	52	16	16	$13.90	$99.00
Mississippi	49	15	14	$17.50	$97.50
Missouri	52	13	15	$17.20	$97.50
Montana	52	16	16	$13.90	$99.00
Nebraska	52	16	16	$13.90	$99.00
Nevada	53	5	15	$12.10	$99.50
New Hampshire	53	18	16	$14.80	$99.50
New Jersey	57	18	18	$14.80	$98.50
New Mexico	55	11	16	$10.40	$97.50
New York	55	15	15	$16.70	$107.50
North Carolina	52	17	16	$14.50	$98.00
North Dakota	52	16	16	$13.90	$99.00
Ohio	58	15	17	$16.60	$98.00
Oklahoma	52	13	15	$16.40	$98.50
Oregon	55	15	17	$14.80	$101.60
Pennsylvania	63	18	17	$15.40	$99.00
Rhode Island	51	14	15	$14.60	$99.50
South Carolina	56	20	15	$15.40	$99.00
South Dakota	52	16	16	$13.90	$99.00
Tennessee	53	15	15	$18.00	$98.00
Texas	56	15	16	$12.10	97.50
Utah	54	14	15	$17.10	$99.50
Vermont	51	14	15	$14.60	$99.50
Virginia	52	17	15	$15.10	$98.00
Washington	55	15	17	$14.80	$101.60
West Virginia	63	18	17	$15.40	$99.00
Wisconsin	57	16	17	$14.10	$99.50
Wyoming	52	16	16	$13.90	$99.00

Sources: CMS, State Data Fact Sheet Source, 2008; The Henry J.Kaiser Family Foundation. Medicare: Part D Plan Characteristics by State, 2008, October 2007.

a. One PDP in Florida covers all generics and some brand name drugs. In other states "some gap coverage" includes plans covering all generics, all preferred generics, or some generics.

When comparing plans it is important to review a number of factors including the breadth of the formulary, the tier particular drugs are placed on, the cost sharing amounts applicable by tier, utilization tools, and the extent of gap coverage. Premiums for 2008 plans with gap coverage generally are twice that for plans without gap coverage.

The average monthly PDP premium, weighted by enrollment was $25.93 in 2006, $27.39 in 2007, and projected to rise to $31.99 in 2008 (presuming beneficiaries do not switch plans).[12]

Part D enrollees typically do not switch plans from year to year. Preliminary analyses suggest that if PDP enrollees do not switch plans between 2007 and 2008, they will likely see a premium increase. One analysis notes that if beneficiaries do not switch plans, three-quarters of those not receiving a low-income subsidy will see a premium increase. Nearly one in five (19%) will see a monthly increase of more than $10. Further one-fourth of enrollees who have not switched from 2006 - 2008 will face a premium increase of at least 50% over the period.[13]

High premium increases are recorded for the two PDPs with the highest enrollment. The average annual premium for AARP's Medicare Rx Plan (offered by UHC-PacifiCare) increased from $316 in 2006 to $388 in 2008. The average annual premium for Humana PDP Standard increased from $114 to $310 in 2008.[14] The increase in United's premium means that it loses its autoenrollment of the low-income subsidy population in 18 out of 34 regions.[15]

COST ESTIMATES

The CBO March 2007 baseline estimates total Part D benefit payments at $47 billion in FY2007, $52.2 billion in FY2008, rising to $140.8 billion in FY2017. (See **Table 8**.)

Table 8. Part D Benefit Payments, Selected Years (estimate in billions of dollars)

Payments	FY2007	FY2008	FY2017
Payments to Plans	27.6	32.1	93.1
Retiree Drug Subsidy	4.1	4.2	4.4
Low-Income Subsidy	15.2	15.9	43.3
Total Benefit Payments	**$47.0**	**$52.2**	**$140.8**

Source: CBO, Fact Sheet for CBO's March 2007 Baseline: Medicare.
Note: Totals may not add due to rounding.

REFERENCES

[1] See CRS Report RL34151, Private Fee for Service (PFFS) Plans: How They Differ from Other Medicare Advantage Plans, by Paulette C. Morgan, Hinda Chaikind, and Holly Stockdale.

[2] The only way that there could be no premium for supplemental benefits is if the plan applied a credit of rebate dollars under the plan's Part C bid against the otherwise applicable premium.

[3] QMBs are aged or disabled persons with incomes at or below the federal poverty level. In 2007, the monthly level is $871 for an individual and $1,161 for a couple (these levels include a monthly $20 disregard for unearned income). Assets must be below $4,000 for an individual and $6,000 for a couple. QMBs are entitled to have their Medicare cost-sharing charges and the Medicare Part B premium paid by the federal-state Medicaid program. Medicaid protection is limited to payment of Medicare cost-sharing charges (i.e., the Medicare beneficiary is not entitled to coverage of Medicaid plan services, such as long term care) unless the individual is otherwise entitled to Medicaid.

[4] SLMBs meet the QMB criteria, except that their income is between 100% and 120% of the federal poverty level. In 2007, the monthly income limits are $1,041 for an individual and $1,389 for a couple. Medicaid protection is limited to payment of the Medicare Part B premium (i.e., the Medicare beneficiary is not entitled to coverage of Medicaid plan services unless the individual is otherwise entitled to Medicaid.

[5] These are persons who meet the QMB criteria, except that their income is between 120% and 135% of poverty. Further, they are not otherwise

eligible for Medicaid. In 2007, the monthly income limit for QI-1 for an individual is $1,169 and for a couple $1,561. Medicaid protection for these persons is limited to payment of the monthly Medicare Part B premium.

[6] CMS, Medicare Expects to Recover $4 Billion from Part D Plans Following 2006 Plan Reconciliation, Press Release, October 5, 2007.
[7] National Association of State Medicaid Directors, 2007 State Perspectives - Medicaid Pharmacy Policies and Practices, November 2007.
[8] The Henry J. Kaiser Family Foundation and Hewitt, Retiree Health Benefits Examined - Findings from the Kaiser/Hewitt 2006 Survey on Retiree Health Benefits, December 2006.
[9] Congressional Budget Office, S. 3, Medicare Prescription Drug Price Negotiation Act of 2007, cost estimate, April 16, 2007.
[10] The Henry J.Kaiser Family Foundation, Overview of Medicare Part D Organizations, Plans and Benefits by Enrollment in 2006 and 2007. November 2007.
[11] Ibid.
[12] The Henry J. Kaiser Family Foundation. Medicare Part D 2008 Data Spotlight: Premiums. November 2007.
[13] Ibid.
[14] Ibid.
[15] Avalere Health LLC. CMS Release of Part D Plan "Landscape" for 2008, September 28, 2007.

INDEX

A

AARP, 72, 75
access, 9, 12, 35, 38, 39, 40, 65
adjustment, 48, 49, 51
administration, 33
adverse event, 44
age, 59
aid, viii, 1, 9, 10
AIDS, 35
Alabama, 69, 73
Alaska, 69, 73
alternative(s), vii, 1, 9, 12, 26, 34, 35, 36, 37, 38, 60, 64
ANOC, 31, 32, 37
anorexia, 33
anti-cancer, 33
anticonvulsant, 35
antidepressant, 35
antineoplastic, 35
antipsychotic, 35
antiretroviral, 35
Arizona, 69, 73
Arkansas, 69, 73
assets, 15, 16, 17, 21, 63
assignment, 21, 22
assumptions, 26
authority, 18, 26, 48
availability, 3, 35
averaging, 19, 48
awareness, 63

B

barbiturates, 33
base year, 56
behavior, 41
benefits, vii, viii, 1, 4, 5, 9, 10, 12, 16, 24, 26, 31, 32, 39, 41, 42, 45, 47, 49, 54, 57, 59, 60, 72, 77
benzodiazepines, 33
biological, 32
bonds, 17
brand name drugs, 30, 74
business, 66

C

California, 69, 73
cancer, 33
catastrophic threshold, 9, 19, 49
chronic diseases, 45
classes, 34, 35, 36
classification, 34
clinical, 34
coinsurance, 10, 20, 29, 36
colds, 33

Colorado, 69, 73
complications, 35
concrete, 64
confidentiality, 40
Congressional Budget Office (CBO), 65, 75, 78
Connecticut, 69, 73
consumer price index (CPI), 15, 16, 20
contracts, 27, 39, 43, 48
coordination, 24, 39
copayment, 10, 29
costs, vii, viii, 1, 6, 9, 10, 18, 20, 24, 26, 33, 44, 45, 47, 48, 49, 50, 51, 54, 56, 59, 60, 64, 65
cost-sharing, vii, viii, 1, 4, 10, 11, 12, 15, 16, 17, 19, 20, 23, 24, 31, 36, 38, 41, 42, 49, 51, 57, 60, 77
coverage, vii, viii, 1, 2, 3, 5, 6, 9, 10, 12, 15, 16, 18, 19, 20, 21, 22, 24, 25, 26, 31, 32, 33, 36, 37, 38, 40, 41, 42, 43, 44, 47, 48, 49, 53, 54, 56, 57, 59, 60, 61, 63, 64, 67, 68, 71, 72, 73, 74, 75, 77
covering, vii, 1, 74
credit, 77
CRS, vii, 77

D

decisions, 34
denial, 41, 42
Department of Defense, 38
disclosure, 40, 65
discounts, 13, 29, 51, 58
disputes, 41
dissatisfaction, 41
distribution, 29, 39, 67, 68
District of Columbia, 25, 69, 73
dosage, 4, 34
doughnut hole, 10, 19
draft, 32
drug interaction, 44
drug manufacturers, 26, 29

drugs, vii, 1, 4, 9, 10, 11, 12, 20, 21, 26, 27, 29, 30, 31, 32, 33, 34, 35, 36, 37, 38, 39, 41, 42, 45, 56, 65, 72, 74, 75

E

education, 39
election, 5
electronic, 45
eligibility criteria, 45
employees, 61
employers, 59, 60, 64
enrollment, vii, 3, 4, 5, 6, 7, 18, 19, 20, 21, 22, 23, 24, 26, 27, 31, 35, 36, 37, 48, 51, 53, 54, 63, 64, 65, 67, 72, 75
erectile dysfunction, 33
erythropoietin, 33
evidence, 31, 34, 42
evidence of coverage (EOC), 31, 32
exclusion, 33, 45
expenditures, 10, 20, 55, 56, 58
extra help, 21

F

family, 10, 17
Federal District Court, 43
Federal Employees Health Benefits (FEHB), 26, 61, 67, 68, 69, 70, 71
federal government, 61
fee(s), 3, 26, 29, 38, 45, 48, 49, 72
fertility, 33
financial support, 17
financing, 26, 49
firms, 61
Food and Drug Administration (FDA), 32, 33, 37, 39
funds, 51

G

generic drug(s), 10, 12, 20, 36, 51, 72
generics, 12, 30, 72, 74

Georgia, 69, 73
government, 50, 57, 61
Government Accountability Office (GAO), 65
grants, 43
groups, 11, 15, 16
growth, 33, 56, 58
growth factor, 56
Guam, 69
guidance, 25
guidelines, 35

H

handling, 39, 40
Hawaii, 69, 73
health, 5, 26, 29, 37, 41, 47, 51, 59, 71
health care, 37
health insurance, 26
health status, 47, 51
hearing, 43
hepatitis, 33
HHS, 61
HIV/AIDS, 35

I

Idaho, 69, 73
Illinois, 69, 73
immunosuppressive drugs, 33
incentives, 44
inclusion, 39, 63
income(s), vii, viii, 1, 2, 5, 7, 10, 11, 15, 16, 17, 19, 18, 20, 21, 22, 23, 24, 35, 47, 51, 53, 54, 57, 63, 64, 68, 72, 73, 75, 77
income determination, 17
Indian, 38, 68
Indian Health Service, 38
Indiana, 69, 73
indication, 32
influenza, 33
initial coverage limit, 9, 12

insulin, 32
insurance, 6, 10, 26, 40, 49
interaction(s), 24, 44
interference, 26
investment, 47

J

judge, 43

K

Kaiser Family Foundation, 61, 71, 74, 78
Kentucky, 70, 73

L

language, 24
law(s), 6, 17, 26, 29, 31, 32, 33, 40, 43, 56, 65
liquid assets, 17
long-term, 37, 38
Louisiana, 70, 73
lower prices, 29
low-income, vii, viii, 1, 2, 5, 7, 10, 11, 15, 16, 18, 20, 21, 22, 23, 24, 35, 47, 51, 53, 54, 57, 63, 64, 68, 72, 75
LTC, 38, 39

M

Maine, 70, 74
management, 27, 29, 35, 36, 37, 42, 44, 58
manufacturer, 33, 37, 58
market(ing), 31, 35, 37, 72
Maryland, 70, 74
Massachusetts, 70, 74
measures, 27, 44
Medicaid, viii, 1, 16, 21, 24, 33, 56, 77, 78

Medicare, vii, viii, 1, 3, 4, 6, 10, 11, 16, 18, 21, 26, 29, 31, 32, 33, 35, 39, 43, 47, 48, 49, 55, 57, 59, 60, 61, 64, 67, 68, 69, 70, 71, 72, 74, 75, 77, 78
Medicare Advantage, vii, 1, 3, 69, 70, 71, 77
Medicare Advantage prescription drug (MA-PD), vii, viii, 1, 3, 9, 15, 16, 19, 21, 24, 38, 48, 54, 59, 60, 61, 63, 67, 69, 70, 71, 72
Medicare Savings Program (MSP), 16, 21, 22, 23
medication, 44, 45
Mexico, 70, 74
military, 5
minerals, 33
Minnesota, 70, 74
Mississippi, 70, 74
Missouri, 70, 74
MMA, vii, 1, 16, 17, 21, 24, 25, 26, 34, 36, 38, 41, 45, 49, 56, 57, 59, 64, 65
Montana, 70, 74

N

national average monthly bid amount, 48, 53
Nebraska, 70, 74
nebulizer, 33
negotiating, 26, 65
negotiation, 26
net price, 29
network, 21, 24, 38, 39, 40, 41, 44
Nevada, 70, 74
New Jersey, 70, 74
New Mexico, 70, 74
New York, 70, 74
North Carolina, 70, 74
nursing, 19

O

Office of Personnel Management, 26

Ohio, 70, 74
Oklahoma, 70, 74
Oregon, 71, 74
organization(s), viii, 3, 11, 12, 21, 23, 26, 27, 31, 72
out-of-pocket, 10, 11, 20, 24, 60, 65
outpatient, 10, 32
oversight, 31

P

PACE, 48
Part D Plans (PDPs), viii, 1, 3, 5, 9, 11, 12, 15, 16, 18, 19, 22, 24, 25, 26, 27, 32, 38, 48, 59, 60, 61, 63, 67, 68, 69, 70, 71, 72, 73, 74, 75, 78
patients, 33
PDP sponsor, 9, 22, 25, 26, 27, 38
penalty, 4, 5, 6, 7, 18, 53, 54
Pennsylvania, 71, 73, 74
per capita, 6, 10, 11, 20, 47, 56, 60
per capita cost, 6
per capita expenditure, 56
performance, 27, 39
permit, 24, 39
pharmaceutical, 10, 24, 29
pharmaceutical benefit managers (PBMs), 29
pharmacies, 21, 26, 29, 36, 37, 38, 39, 40, 45, 65
pharmacists, 27, 34, 36, 44
physicians, 33, 34, 36, 44
pilot study, 45
planning, 25
play, 63
population, 15, 35, 56, 57, 63, 75
poverty, viii, 1, 11, 15, 16, 17, 18, 19, 20, 21, 77
premium(s), vii, viii, 1, 4, 6, 11, 12, 15, 16, 17, 18, 20, 21, 22, 23, 24, 29, 47, 48, 51, 53, 54, 55, 57, 60, 63, 64, 65, 72, 73, 75, 77, 78
prescription drug plans, vii, 1, 53

Index

Prescription Drug, Improvement, and Modernization Act, vii, 1
price index, 15
prices, 9, 12, 29, 36, 65
procedures, 20, 37, 40
profit(s), 47, 49
program, vii, 1, 3, 4, 6, 9, 10, 16, 18, 20, 29, 35, 38, 44, 45, 49, 51, 55, 58, 61, 63, 65, 77
proxy, 56
public, 5, 29
Public Health Service (PHS), 32
Puerto Rico, 71

Q

QMBs, 16, 77
quality assurance, 44

R

random, 20, 21
random assignment, 21
range, 16, 36, 50, 73
real estate, 17
rebates, 13, 29, 30, 51, 54, 56, 58, 65
reconciliation, 49, 51
reduction, 56
reflection, 51
regional, 18, 19, 23, 38
regulations, 16, 17, 26, 31
reinsurance, 26, 47, 49, 51, 53
renal disease, 33
resolution, 27
resources, 15, 16, 17, 45
retail, 29, 38, 39, 58
retiree(s), 5, 59, 60, 61
revenue, 47
Rhode Island, 71, 74
risk, vii, 1, 25, 26, 33, 40, 44, 47, 48, 49, 50, 51
risk profile, 25, 47
rural areas, 39, 65

S

safety, 34, 36
sales, 31
savings, 17, 29, 50, 56, 58, 64, 65
savings account, 17
scientific, 34
security, 55, 57
selecting, 64
sharing, vii, viii, 1, 4, 10, 11, 12, 15, 16, 17, 19, 20, 23, 24, 31, 36, 38, 39, 41, 42, 47, 49, 51, 57, 60, 75, 77
SLMBs, 16, 77
smoking cessation, 33
social security, 17, 21, 55, 57
solvency, 26
South Carolina, 71, 74
South Dakota, 71, 74
spouse, 4, 17, 59
stages, 20
standards, 17, 26, 34, 37, 38, 39, 44, 45
state laws, 40
strength, 34
subgroups, 15
subsidy(ies), vii, viii, 1, 2, 6, 7, 10, 11, 13, 15, 16, 17, 18, 19, 20, 21, 22, 23, 24, 26, 33, 47, 48, 49, 51, 53, 54, 55, 57, 59, 60, 61, 63, 64, 67, 68, 75
supplemental, 12, 24, 25, 47, 54, 77
Supplemental Security Income (SSI), 16, 21, 22, 23
supply, 37, 38, 39
systems, 34, 44, 45

T

taxes, 59
telephone, 27
Tennessee, 71, 74
Texas, 71, 74
therapeutic, 34, 36, 44
therapy, 35, 37, 44
third party, 60

threshold(s), 9, 10, 11, 19, 36, 49, 50, 64
time frame, 43
transactions, 45
transition, 18, 19, 37, 38, 56
transplant, 33
Treasury, 55
TROOP, 10, 11, 24, 60
trust fund, 55, 57

U

uniform, 45, 53
unions, 59, 60
United States, 34, 69
urban areas, 39
urbanized, 27
Utah, 71, 74

V

vaccines, 32, 33
variation, 26, 48
Vermont, 71, 74
Virginia, 71, 73, 74
vitamins, 33

W

wait times, 27
Washington, 71, 74
weight gain, 33
weight loss, 33
wholesalers, 29
Wisconsin, 71, 74